SWIMS
C20348732

AF606627

WITHDRAWN

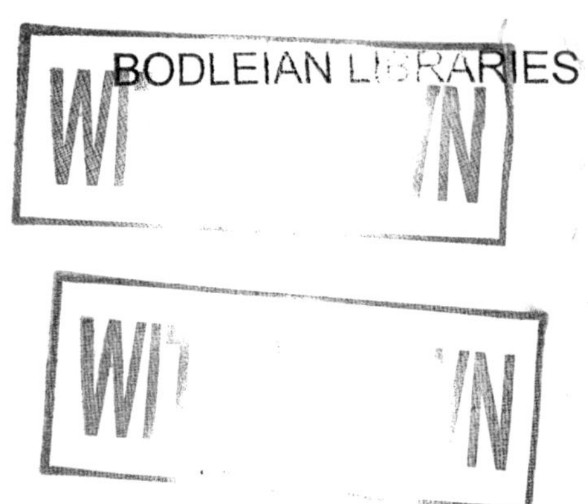

THE VERY STUFF OF GENERAL PRACTICE

Edited by
Philippa Moreton

Radcliffe Medical Press

Radcliffe Medical Press Ltd
18 Marcham Road, Abingdon, Oxon OX14 1AA

British Library Cataloguing in Publication Data

A catalogue record for this book is available from the British Library.

ISBN 1 85775 390 9

Typeset by Advance Typesetting Ltd, Oxfordshire
Printed and bound by Biddles Ltd, Guildford and King's Lynn

Dedication

This book is dedicated to John Hasler on his retirement from the post of Director of Postgraduate Education for General Practice at Oxford after 25 years, and on his retirement from full-time general practice. Whether we came to know him as his students, protégés, colleagues or, strictly speaking, subordinates, we all now write as his friends. He has touched us all. We have worked with him, laughed a great deal together and, though a naïve observer may not have recognised it, we have even disagreed with him – though usually not for long.

The book is a Festschrift, celebrating John's contribution to general practice, which has been enormous. Through his work in Oxford, he has been associated with many of the most innovative and influential initiatives in general practice teaching of the last two decades. The list is long and includes teaching the consultation using video-recordings, approval of training practices through peer review visits, the core curriculum for the teaching of general practice at postgraduate level and many others.

In this context, it is imperative to understand how he has been able to do so much. The answer is: through others. John's contribution has been that of a real leader. He has rarely initiated alone but rather has operated through an impressive group of colleagues who he has recruited, nurtured and developed. He has always had a keen sense of the current most pressing issues in his field and has focused the attention of his team repeatedly on these matters. He has invited their contributions and initiatives, taken a full (peer) role in the discussions and acted as an evaluator of the ideas proposed. He has been remarkably perceptive in recognising solutions as they have emerged from the dialogue and has then found the resources, both intellectual and financial, to help support the initiative. He has acted as coach, mentor and cheerleader and has never let bureaucracy stand in the way of progress.

I have been the beneficiary of this style of leadership, if I may be permitted a personal note. I arrived in Oxford knowing no one, but wanting to conduct my doctoral research on the subject of doctor–patient communication. I had been advised by my doctoral supervisor that my ideas were interesting but that 'the medics will never let you in to their world'. I was introduced by my college doctor to John Hasler, the Regional Adviser in General Practice. Within weeks the research had begun and I was a welcome member of the Oxford Region's Course Organiser group. Within twelve months our teaching on the consultation had become established and three years later we started to write '*The consultation*'. The turning point was meeting John and his willingness to encourage a complete unknown, trusting his own judgement that something good could be made to happen in this way.

He has played a full role also in the profession beyond the Oxford Region. In the Royal College of General Practitioners, he served as both Secretary to Council and its Chairman. He was a member of many working parties and committees including the *What sort of doctor?* working party and he was an examiner for many years. He has inspected countless practices and courses for the Joint Committee for Postgraduate Training in General Practice both in the UK and around the world.

He has authored and edited many books and papers and the list is far too long to be included here. He has served as a distinguished member of the editorial board of journals and book series. He has presented honour lectures around the world. He has received an OBE for his services to general practice education. He has even found time to complete an MD because he felt it was important for him to do so.

Despite all of these achievements, I suspect it will be his contribution as a leader that has been most significant and unusual. Few people have been able to equal his ability to make things happen with and through others, to build a loyal and high quality team, and to develop talent unselfishly.

Those who love general practice owe him a debt of gratitude. Those of us who have worked with him understand the respect he is owed. Those of us who count him as a friend feel even more and he knows.

Thanks John.

David Pendleton
January 1999

Contents

List of contributors

Peter Havelock General Practitioner, Wooburn Green, Buckinghamshire, and Associate Adviser to General Practice, Oxford Deanery.

Jacqueline Hayden General Practitioner, Unsworth, Lancashire, and Dean of Postgraduate Medical Education in the North West Region.

Lynne Hobden-Clarke Management Consultant.

Jennifer King Chartered Psychologist and Management Consultant and Director of the Edgecumbe Consulting Group Ltd.

Ann-Louise Kinmonth General Practitioner and Professor of General Practice, Cambridge University.

Martin Lawrence General Practitioner, Chipping Norton, Oxfordshire, and University Lecturer, Department of Primary Health Care, Oxford University.

David Metcalfe Professor of General Practice and Senior Coordinator for Curricular Change, Manchester University Medical School (retired).

David Pendleton Chartered Psychologist and Management Consultant, and Director and Founder of the Edgecumbe Consulting Group Ltd.

Mike Pringle General Practitioner, Collingham, Nottinghamshire, and Professor of General Practice, University of Nottingham.

Theo Schofield General Practitioner, Shipston-on-Stour, Warwickshire, and University Lecturer, Department of Primary Health Care, Oxford University. Formerly Associate Adviser in the Oxford Region.

Preface

This book was conceived and written as a tribute to John Hasler on the occasion of his retirement from general practice and Director of Postgraduate General Practice Education, a post he had held for 25 years. Each author in this book has made their own special contribution to general practice but each of them has reason to be grateful to John Hasler as a friend and mentor. It is a testament to his outstanding ability to nurture and develop others that there are so many eminent people who have succeeded with his encouragement and support.

Each author was asked to write about a subject related to general practice that they cared deeply about. The result is a remarkable collection of chapters looking at a wide range of important general practice issues that can be grouped under headings of teaching, learning and leadership.

These contributions have been written by professionals who have all contributed to the national and international debate on their chosen subject. They are particularly valuable because they capture the enthusiasm and commitment of each author to their area of expertise in a way that brings the subject alive. They also bring a unique historical perspective to their chapters, demonstrating the development of their chosen subject within general practice over the years, and in many cases outlining the challenges ahead. Many authors have reviewed the literature on their chosen subject and there are many references and annotated bibliographies

The topics covered in this book are all to do with professional and practice development and quality improvement. The government White Paper *A first class service* has set the development of quality at the heart of the new NHS and primary care will be required to develop clinical governance, which is accountability for improving and safeguarding high standards of care by using the principles of evidence-based practice and risk management. In addition, the Paper states that 'life-long learning is an investment in quality', and each clinician will have to develop and use personal learning plans. The challenges for primary care are huge and this book will provide much of the background and current thinking about the development of practices and individuals just at the time when this becomes a high priority for primary care groups.

This book will be relevant for all members of the primary care team including doctors, nurses and practice managers. Individuals will be able to pick out one chapter to read easily at one sitting.

Many of the thoughts and opinions of the authors are similar. This is not surprising considering that they all share the same mentor, John Hasler, to whom this book is dedicated and who, through his ability to share his vision and values, has ensured that the work he started is continuing.

There can be no greater tribute to a man than that.

Philippa Moreton
January 1999

1

The consultation: an approach to learning and teaching revisited

Theo Schofield and Peter Havelock

Outline

- The approach to the consultation developed in Oxford and published in 1984 included tasks that defined an effective patient-centred consultation, and a learner-centred method of teaching.
- Since then, this approach has been developed and disseminated, particularly by workshops for teachers, and incorporated into the assessment of vocational training for general practice.
- New research and other approaches to teaching have also been developed in other centres and these are described.

Introduction

The consultation: an approach to learning and teaching was published by Oxford University Press in 1984.[1] This chapter describes the ways in which the ideas it contains were originally developed, how they were diffused into medical teaching and practice, and how the concepts of effective consulting and teaching have continued to develop since then.

The principles behind the approach

The approach was the result of a collaboration between David Pendleton, a social psychologist who was conducting research in doctor–patient communication, and three general practitioners with particular interests and responsibilities for vocational training for general practice. The book was the result of close working and cooperation between all the authors whose variety of backgrounds, teaching, research, psychology, an interest in anthropology, Balint training, and experience of consulting with patients, blended together to form the approach that we took to the consultation. There were a number of principles that were agreed that guided not only the writing of the book, but also the running of the teaching courses and the strategy for the implementation of the ideas in practice. Those principles were:

- All people have ideas and concerns about their health
- Most people wish to have involvement in their healthcare
- People's understanding of their health governs their health behaviour
- Doctors have a wider role in the consultation than just the diagnosis and management of disease, such as health promotion, modifying health-seeking behaviour, and encouraging patient autonomy
- People need to base new learning on their current understanding, so their understanding has to be sought before teaching occurs
- Nearly all doctors have a range of sophisticated communication skills, although these are sometimes not used in their consultations
- Everyone can improve their communication skills
- Learning experiences should match the messages in the teaching (i.e. patient-centred consulting needs to be taught with a learner-centred approach)
- Different people learn in different ways so teaching needs to have different methods, levels of abstraction and sources, but the message needs to be consistent

- There are three stages of effective skill development:
  1. A clear idea of what is to be learnt
  2. Opportunity to practise with feedback on performance
  3. Time and a strategy to get the lessons into routine performance
- People develop more effectively when they have a clear idea of their strengths, a clear idea of what they need to improve, and how that change can be achieved.

Ingredients of the approach

The approach to learning and teaching the consultation had two principal ingredients. The first was the development of a *model of an effective consultation* which included not only the clinical task of establishing the nature of the patient's problem and its aetiology, but also the patient-centred tasks of exploring the patient's ideas, concerns and expectations about the problem and its management, and sharing understanding, decisions and responsibility with patients. Secondly, it described a *method of teaching* which was based on observing how effectively a doctor achieved these tasks in a consultation, and giving feedback that identified his or her strengths and helped the doctor to consider alternative ways in which they could become more effective.

There were a number of parallels between these processes. They described a patient-centred style of consulting in which the central purpose was to identify and to meet the patient's needs, and the teaching as being learner-centred in that the learner was encouraged to identify his or her own strengths and weaknesses and to set the agenda for his or her teaching. They also described the consultation as part of a cycle of care in which patients' understanding and ability to manage their own health were enhanced at each consultation, and the central purpose of the teaching was to help learners to understand their own consultation style and the ways in which they could develop and become more effective.

The 'hardware' element of the package was a set of tools to help teachers use this approach including a consultation map, a rating scale, and 'rules' to control the feedback process. These were designed to make feedback more effective, by identifying and reinforcing the learner's strengths, as well as encouraging peer learning, and also more acceptable than the critical approach usually experienced in medical education.

Dissemination of the approach

Diffusion is the process by which an innovation is communicated through certain channels over time among the members of a social system.[2] The factors that can influence the rate at which a new practice is adopted, or whether it is adopted at all, include the nature of the innovation itself, the relationship between its proponents and the potential adopters, the characteristics of the adopters, and the social system within which diffusion takes place.

The nature of the innovation

The characteristics of an innovation that determine its rate of adoption are its:

- Relative advantage over existing practice
- Compatibility with existing values and practice
- Complexity and difficulty to understand and use
- Trialability, the degree to which it can be tried on a limited basis
- Observability to others.

There is no question that trainers believed that the approach to teaching fulfilled these characteristics. The importance of the doctor–patient relationship as the core of general practice was part of the shared values of GP teachers, being patient- and learner-centred felt right, and the structured methods of observation and feedback were found to be preferable to the critical comments that often came from comparing the learner with oneself!

Reducing the degree of complexity and threat, allowing trainers to try out the approach in a protected environment, and giving them the opportunity to observe others doing so were also achieved by the trainers' workshops described below.

The difficulty, which we will discuss more fully later in the chapter, was, and remains, with the approach to consulting in practice, which can be seen as less advantageous and more risky than more traditional styles learnt at medical school. Exploring patients' ideas and concerns can be seen as time consuming, patients vary widely in their desire and expectation to be involved in decisions about their care. Given the opportunity, patients may express views that are assertive or critical, and there are two small but widely quoted studies that purport to show that patients prefer an authoritative style of doctoring.[3,4] These reservations continue to be relevant.

The proponents and adopters

The approach to the consultation was developed over a number of years through a process of active debate and development among the authors, and testing the acceptability and feasibility of the ideas by presenting them to a series of teachers' courses. This was a very important and valuable part of the process, as a much wider range of views were able to be included, albeit only those of trainers, and the eventual publication reflected this consensus. However, once the ideas were crystallised and published there was a danger that they could become set in 'tablets of stone'.

As well as improving the product this method of development reduced the distance between the innovators and the adopters, and created a degree of ownership of the ideas among a body of credible opinion leaders in their local trainers' groups who acted as advocates. Trainers, particularly those who go on new courses, are likely to be early adopters of new ideas, whereas late adopters are more likely to be isolated and have less positive attitudes to, and experience of, change.

The social system

As well as the relatively informal networks of courses and workshops, trainers are also part of a structured accreditation and re-accreditation system of training practice assessments. Once the majority of trainers have adopted any innovation it is possible to include encouragement or even sanctions to ensure that any laggards comply. Thus, over the years, trainers have been asked to show one of their own consultations to the visiting assessors, to demonstrate how they teach, and more recently, to ensure that all their registrars are prepared for their summative assessments of their own recorded consultations. There is no comparable system of encouragement or assessment for GPs not involved in training.

In the Oxford Region the message has also been reinforced by including sessions on the consultation in the introductory and day release courses for registrars, thus creating consumer demand for teaching in practice.

Teaching the teachers

The most important aspect of the activities to promote communication skills teaching in practice has been the workshops for teachers in the majority of regions in the UK. The Oxford Region workshops have been attended by over 1000 GP trainers. In addition, a number of regions have adapted the approach and are running their own workshops. The workshops that are now provided last three days and are usually residential. The key elements in the programme are:

Day 1

- Establishing the participant's previous experience of communication skills teaching and their own expectations of the course and what they wish to achieve. These discussions take place in small groups of up to six doctors and these groups then have the opportunity of meeting these individual needs over the next three days of the course. This is deliberately paralleling the process of patient-centred consulting and learner-centred teaching that the workshop aims to promote

- The evidence and rationale that underpin the approach to the consultation are presented, and other approaches to analysing and teaching the consultation that the trainers may wish to explore and use are also described

- The process of observing, describing, and giving feedback on consultations using the tutor's tapes as examples is then described and rehearsed. At the end of this first day, the trainers are therefore provided with an explicit model of what it is they are trying to teach both for the consultation and for their teaching.

Day 2
The second day is spent in small groups with each member of the group in turn conducting a consultation with a simulated patient in front of the group and then receiving feedback from them. This has a number of functions. The group has the opportunity of rehearsing the process of observing and giving feedback on consultations and the group leader can participate in the process and can help group members develop their skills during the day. The individual doctors have the opportunity of experiencing feedback from colleagues and learning from it, and by explicitly identifying effective skills and strategies in each consultation, the group has the opportunity to learn a wider repertoire of effective consultation behaviours so that they are able to offer their learners' alternative approaches rather than just their own. The simulated patients play a very important part during the day. Apart from acting roles that can be chosen to provide a variety of teaching points, they are also available to give feedback in the group, first, while they remain in role and then as co-teachers drawing on their previous experience.

Day 3
On the third day, each member of the group is invited to watch a pre-recorded consultation by another member of the group and then to give feedback to that doctor. The rest of the group do not participate in this feedback but instead observe the teaching and give feedback to the teacher on its effectiveness. This means that each member of the group has the opportunity to rehearse, as an individual, what they learnt in the group on the previous day. The workshop therefore also exemplifies the three ingredients of effective skills teaching, an explicit model of what is to be learnt, opportunities for practice, and observation and feedback.

Finally, the members of the course are invited to write a personal action plan of how they intend to use and develop what they have learnt during the course and then they participate in its final evaluation.

Evaluation

The evaluation reports that have been written at the end of each workshop have helped the continuing development of the course structure. However, probably the most influential method of evaluation has been the number of occasions on which outside observers have been invited to take part in the course and then to make recommendations for change. The outcome of the course in improving teachers' skills has been evaluated by inviting them to write down the comments that they would make to the doctor having seen the same pre-recorded consultation at the beginning and end of the workshop and rating these comments on the extent to which they are drawn from the tasks and whether they follow a sequence of strengths, weaknesses, and recommendations. This evaluation is also positive.

In 1989, the results of a controlled study were published comparing the patients' perceptions of the consultations of teachers attending the course with those of matched controls.[5] There were small but significant changes in the extent that patients felt they had been involved in decisions and given more responsibility, but they also became more concerned!

What has not been carried out is either to evaluate the effect of the course on the teaching done by trainers or, more importantly, its effectiveness in helping their learners' consultations.

The problem of evaluation

Part of the problem is that since the early days of this innovation, communication skills teaching, it has been rapidly changing and developing, and although participant and observer evaluations were extremely valuable during the first stages, embarking on a more formal outcome study in a controlled design can impede further development. There is a later stage when the innovation is so widely adopted that a controlled study becomes very difficult, but there was undoubtedly a window of opportunity between these two stages when the piloting and development was nearing completion when the next stage of dissemination could be done in a controlled study, either before or after, or randomised. However, it has not been the prevailing ethos within postgraduate education for general practice to expect rigorous evaluation and we relied much more heavily on face validity, acceptability, and anecdotal accounts of benefit to decide whether new innovations should be adopted. This is exacerbated by the separation of postgraduate departments and university departments of general practice in almost all parts of the country so that postgraduate education has not been exposed as much to the ethos of research and publication, and has not had ready access to people with those skills. Also, the type of people who enjoy and are adept at developing new ideas and teaching them (like the authors!) may not have the skills, the patience, or even the time to do good quality research. This may change with growing emphasis on evidence-based medicine, and will be greatly helped by much closer relationships between undergraduate and postgraduate departments.

Evidence of effective implementation

The extent to which this approach has been adopted in vocational training is, however, known. In 1995, a questionnaire was sent to all the trainers, course organisers and advisers in the Oxford Region seeking their views, use of, and blocks to consultation teaching. 97% of trainers in the region had easy access to a video camera and over 60% of trainees had their consultations reviewed four times a year or more. The block to effective teaching was time rather than lack of skill or belief in the need for consultation skill teaching. A similar survey in the West Midlands found that 93% of trainers used video-recording for teaching and that our framework was the most commonly used assessment tool.[6] The introduction of the observation of recorded consultations as a method of assessment in both the Royal College of General Practitioners examination and in summative assessment, and the fact that the criteria used are derived from the tasks, are key markers of the general acceptance of this work.[7]

However, the two research studies that have been conducted based on recorded consultations by volunteer GPs, a proportion of whom were trainers in the Oxford Region, have shown great variation in the degree to which the tasks were achieved in those consultations.[8,9] In this, as in many other areas, the challenge remains to bridge the gap between theory and evidence on the one hand, and actual practice on the other.

Other descriptions of the consultation approach

The approach to learning and teaching was based on earlier descriptions of the consultation and on David Pendleton's review of the available evidence on doctor–patient communication.[10] Since then, the literature has grown substantially and some other approaches have had a major influence on current thinking.

Meetings between experts

David Tuckett and his colleagues described the consultation as a meeting between two experts, one in medicine and one in their own lives and illness, and they make the case for the importance of sharing ideas between them.[11] The research that they undertook was undoubtedly the most comprehensive and rigorous of any undertaken on doctor–patient communication in the UK. Because their results were published in a book rather than in separate papers in scientific journals, their results are far less frequently quoted than they deserve to be. Their core messages were:

- Doctors frequently give patients information about the diagnosis and management and future prevention of their problems, but rarely seek the patients' ideas about them, and even more rarely give their explanations in ways that actually react or interact with the patients' own ideas
- Patients do retain the majority of the important messages that their doctor intended to give them, but the most frequent explanation of why they were not retained was that they were couched in language or used ideas that the patient did not understand

The patient-centred clinical method

The Department of Family Practice in London, Ontario, led by Ian McWhinney and Moira Stewart first published a description of the patient-centred clinical method in 1985.[12] This describes the function of a medical interview as exploring two agendas, the doctor's related to the symptoms and disease, and the patient's including his or her concerns, fears, and illness experience, and then integrating both. They have since described six interactive components in such a consultation which share many of the characteristics of the tasks:

1 Exploring both the disease and the illness experience
   - differential diagnosis
   - dimensions of illness (ideas, feelings, expectations and effects)
2 Understanding the whole person
   - the person (life history and personal development)
   - the context
3 Finding common ground regarding management
   - problems and priorities
   - goals of treatment
   - roles of doctor and patient in management
4 Incorporating prevention and health promotion
   - health enhancement
   - risk reduction
   - early detection of disease
   - ameliorating effects of disease
5 Enhancing the doctor–patient relationship
   - characteristics of the therapeutic relationship
   - sharing power
   - caring and healing relationship
   - self-awareness
   - transference and countertransference
6 Being realistic
   - time
   - resources
   - team building.

In 1995, Moira Stewart and colleagues published *Patient-centered medicine*,[13] which described the development of these concepts and ways in which they can be taught and evaluated, and the research evidence that supported them. They worked independently over the same period as the group in Oxford, but both are very happy to acknowledge the large amount of common ground that there is between them.

The ethical imperative for patient-centred care was eloquently described by Ian McWhinney in his chapter on transforming the clinical method.[14]

> Our modern dedication to instrumental knowledge requires that any change in what we do be justified by its effects. Does the patient-centered method improve patients' health? There is good evidence that it does. But I believe we are mistaken if we make this its justification. Some things are good in themselves. The justification of the patient-centered method is its moral basis.
>
> Medicine has perennial moral problems, two of which are particularly serious in the present age: insensitivity to suffering and abuse of power. The distancing produced by our abstractions makes us especially prone to the first; our greatly enhanced prognostic and therapeutic power makes us especially liable to the second. Reforming our clinical method has at its deepest level a moral purpose: a restoration of the balance between thinking and feeling and a renunciation, or at least a sharing, of the enormous power modern technology has given us.

The inner consultation

Roger Neighbour's book aims to help doctors increase their awareness and consult more effectively and describes five stages that take place at the consultation.[15]

1 Connecting

2 Summarising

3 Handover

4 Safety-netting

5 Housekeeping.

Although the stages of connecting and handing over were similarly patient-centred to the tasks, the task of safety-netting, ensuring that plans are made to catch any unexpected future developments, is missing from the Oxford approach. Housekeeping and developing the doctor's ability to recognise and cope with their own feelings during and after consultations are also very important parts of becoming a more effective doctor, but are not part of the approach that was originally described.

Research support for the approach

The cycle of care was originally developed by David Pendleton as a way of describing the research teacher in doctor–patient communication.[10] A large majority of the studies correlated aspects of the patient, doctor or the setting with behaviour in the consultation or correlations between these factors and outcomes. He classified outcomes as *immediate,* such as memory for information, satisfaction, changes in concern, *intermediate* outcomes, particularly compliance and *long-term* changes in health. Since then, the literature has continued to grow. More recently, a meta-analysis of over 60 papers correlated aspects of behaviour in the consultation with the outcomes of memory, satisfaction, and compliance.[16]

This approach, however, has substantial limitations. It is likely there are confounding variables, such as the characteristics of the patient or their problem, that lead to the variations in behaviour in the consultation and in subsequent outcome. Secondly, the correlations in most of the studies reviewed by Roter are in fact quite small and fail to explain the extent of the variation of outcome. Finally, the value of satisfaction as an outcome has been questioned in the light of other evidence which shows that approaches that are less directive and encourage patient involvement may threaten immediate satisfaction but can result in improved long-term health of the patient.

The most rigorous evidence in support of expanding patient involvement has been provided by a series of randomised controlled trials conducted by Greenfield, Kaplan and Weare.[17] In their studies, patients with chronic diseases were given more information about their condition and encouraged to ask more questions and take a more active part in their subsequent consultations with their physician. The outcomes were not only that the consultations themselves included more questions and more challenging statements by the patients, but also improved physiological measures and reduced functional limitations were achieved, when compared to groups of control patients who had not been subjected to the intervention.

Lars Lassen[18] demonstrated that the degree of achievement of patient-centred tasks can predict the likelihood of patients complying with their doctor's advice, and working with him the authors were able to replicate this in a larger sample of British GPs.[9] This work has helped to establish the reliability and validity of the approach of rating the effectiveness of consultations on task achievement.

The more recent evidence that supports patient-centred communication has been reviewed by Stewart[19] and Putnam and Lipkin,[20] but contains a very limited number of controlled trials. To be persuasive in medical settings, research in doctor–patient communication needs to match the rigour that would be applied to other medical interventions. There is therefore a need for more controlled trials if their results are to be seen as relevant by teachers and practitioners, and they need to be conducted in healthcare systems similar to their own.

Development of communication skills teaching in medical schools

There has been an expansion of communication skills teaching in medical schools in the UK and this has been supported and encouraged by successive reports by the Education Committee of the General Medical Council. Teachers have largely been drawn from general practice, psychiatry and behavioural science, and many innovative approaches from different medical schools have been described. However, the teaching is usually provided by general practitioners, psychiatrists, or behavioural scientists and is often quite separate from other clinical teaching. It is therefore understandable if medical students come to understand that 'real' doctors take histories from patients and only later in their professional lives rediscover the value of listening to them.

In introducing communication skills teaching during the first clinical year in Oxford there has been a continued mismatch between the teaching and the communication that the students are actually observing. Although all doctors in hospital, particularly junior staff, are subjected to considerable and continuing pressures on their time, there is still a lack of clarity about how history-taking and patient-centred consulting can be combined successfully. Interaction issues are rarely discussed or taught explicitly and students' communication skills are not observed or assessed either informally during their clinical attachments, or formally in examinations.

Today, students starting to learn the practice of clinical medicine have to cope with many mixed messages from their clinical and communication skills teachers: being asked to 'take a history' from which they are meant to be able to provide a differential diagnosis, while observing practising doctors being selective and generating and testing hypotheses; learning a list of questions to be asked, and then being taught to ask open questions and remain silent; and being taught to explore the patients' ideas and concerns, and then never being asked to include these in their case presentations.

There is a need to develop a coherent model of a clinical interview that can be taught to clinical medical students by both clinical and communication skills teachers. This model should help the student become clinically effective as a practising doctor, and also be patient-centred, meeting the needs of their patients.

This model must include the tasks that are to be achieved, the strategies that can be employed, and the skills that are required. It is also necessary to consider the problems and situations in which the student and young doctor will be involved and are expected to be competent.

As well as helping the student to learn, such a model could also be the basis for the assessment of student progress during their clinical studies. When every student is routinely asked when presenting a patient –

- What does the patient understand about his or her problem?
- What is the patient worried or concerned about?
- How is the problem affecting his or her life?
- What would the patient like us to do for him or her?

– we will know we have arrived.

Developing the concept of evidence-based patient choice

The nature of the relationship between doctors and patients and their respective roles in making decisions about treatment has been the subject of intense ethical debate around the meaning of 'informed consent'. Some protagonists argue for patient autonomy and fully informed choice and others maintain that the doctor continues to have the responsibility for making medical decisions which patients can choose or decline to follow.

When offered a choice between the doctor or the patient making choices about treatment, a substantial proportion of patients say that they prefer their doctor to decide. This preference varies with the severity of the condition, the patient's educational background, and whether they believe they or their doctor is in control of their health.[5] However, this is a false dichotomy and given the choice of mutual decision-making the strongest preferences, in an Australian report, were for 'You and your doctor together' and 'Your doctor after getting information'.[21] Further exploration found that the factors valued most by patients were information exchange and the nature of the relationship, and that patients were happy to accept doctors' decisions if they felt the doctor understood them as a person, had listened to their views, and explained the reasons for the decisions that had been made.

The concept of 'evidence-based patient choice' has been described by Tony Hope.[22] He explores the difficulty inherent in synthesising the currently fashionable concept of evidence-based medicine with its implication that there is a correct or preferred treatment and the ethical perspective of patients' choice. In considering how this can be resolved in the consultation he identifies the issues of the quality of the information the patient is given, how it is framed, how it is understood, how patients are enabled to make choices, and how the nature of the doctor–patient relationship may change in the future.

The future

The above issues are central to any discussion about the future direction of communication skills training. On the one hand, we have the ethical imperative and the growing body of evidence to support patient-centred approaches to consulting. On the other, we have the evidence that this approach has not been fully adopted in practice, and the doctors' understandable reservations about time, acceptability to patients, and whether it can be done effectively.

The social climate is changing with less automatic acceptance of professional authority, and rising consumerism, and a growing range of alternative sources of information for patients. These can be seen as opportunities or as threats by practitioners. If we are to achieve real movement and avoid conflict we must remember the lessons we have learnt about successful diffusion of innovation. We must ensure that patient-centred consulting and patient partnerships are seen as compatible with, and have advantages over, existing practice. We need to ensure that accessing new sources of information by both doctors and patients is easy, understandable, and not disruptive. Training, the opportunity to experiment in a safe supportive environment, and to observe others, needs to be provided. Above all, we need trusted and credible opinion leaders within the profession. There is still work to be done.

Summary

- Teaching communication skills using video-recording and structured feedback is an innovation that has been successfully diffused throughout vocational training for general practice in the UK.
- There is a growing body of evidence to support the effectiveness of patient-centred consulting, but less evidence to show that this happens in practice.

References

1 Pendleton D, Schofield T, Tate P and Havelock P (1984) *The consultation: an approach to learning and teaching.* Oxford University Press.

2 Rogers E (1983) *Diffusion of innovations.* The Free Press, New York.

3 Savage R and Armstrong D (1990) Effect of a general practitioner's consulting style on patients' satisfaction: a controlled study. *British Medical Journal,* **301**: 968–70.

4 Thomas K B (1987) General practice consultations: is there any point in being positive? *British Medical Journal*, **294**:1200–2.

5 Arnson P, Makoul G, Pendleton D and Schofield T (1989) Patients' perceptions of medical encounters in Great Britain: variations with health loci of control and sociodemographic factors. *Health Communication*, **1**:75–95.

6 Field S (1985) The use of video recording in general practice education: a survey of trainers in the West Midlands region. *Education for General Practice*, **6**:49–58.

7 Campbell L, Howie J and Murray T (1995) Use of videotaped consultations in summative assessment of trainees in general practice. *British Journal of General Practice*, **45**:137–41.

8 Makoul G, Arnson P and Schofield T (1995) Health promotion in primary care: physician-patient communication and decision making about prescribed medications. *Social Science and Medicine*, **41**:1241–54.

9 Lassen C, Schofield T and Havelock P (in press) The reliability and validity of consultation measures.

10 Pendleton D (1983) Doctor–patient communication: a review. In: D Pendleton and J Hasler (eds) *Doctor–patient communication*. Academic Press, London.

11 Tuckett D, Boulton M, Olson C and Williams A (1985) *Meetings between experts: an approach to sharing medical ideas in medical consultations*. Tavistock, London.

12 Levenstein J, McCracken E, McWhinney I, Stewart M and Brown J (1986) The patient-centred clinical method. 1. A model for the doctor–patient interaction in family medicine. *Family Practice*, **3**:24–30.

13 Stewart M, *et al.* (1995) *Patient-centered medicine: transforming the clinical method*. Sage, Thousand Oaks.

14 McWhinney I (1995) Why we need a new clinical method. In: M Stewart *et al.* (eds) *Patient-centered medicine: transforming the clinical method*. Sage, Thousand Oaks.

15 Neighbour R (1987) *The inner consultation*. MTP Press, Lancaster.

16 Hall J, Roter D and Katz N (1988) Meta-analysis of correlates of provider behaviour in medical encounters. *Medical Care*, **26**:657–75.

17 Greenfield S, Kaplan S and Ware J (1985) Expanding patient involvement in care: effects on patient outcomes. *Annals of Internal Medicine*, **102**:520–8.

18 Lassen L (1991) Connections between the quality of consultations and patient compliance in general practice. *Family Practice*, **8**:154–60.

19 Stewart M A (1995) Effective physician–patient communication and health outcomes: a review. *Canadian Medical Association Journal*, **152**:1423–33.

20 Putnam S M and Lipkin M (1995) The patient centered interview: research support. In: M Lipkin, S M Putnam and A Lazare (eds) *The medical interview*. Springer, New York.

21 Smith D, Garko M, Bennett K, Irwin H and Schofield T (1994) Patient preferences for delegation and participation: cross national support for mutuality. *Australian Journal of Communication*, **21**:86–108.

22 Hope T (1996) *Evidence-based patient choice*. The King's Fund, London.

Further reading

1 Lipkin M, Putnam S M and Lazare A (eds) (1995) *The medical interview*. Springer, New York.
A comprehensive text for reference which includes an extensive bibliography.

2 Stewart M, *et al.* (1995) *Patient-centered medicine: transforming the clinical method*. Sage, Thousand Oaks.
A classic that describes the work of a unit that has tackled the research, teaching and ethical issues involved in patient-centred care.

3 Tuckett D, Boulton M, Olson C and Williams A (1985) *Meetings between experts: an approach to sharing medical ideas in medical consultations*. Tavistock, London.
A somewhat dense book that contains many important ideas and research findings. Well worth the effort!

2

Leading peers

David Pendleton

Outline

General practice is not hierarchical. It is a flat world of peers who are organised into partnerships. There are no appointed leaders, yet leadership is called for to enhance standards and advance the profession. This chapter describes approaches to leadership that can work in a flat world. These are models of leadership that work through clarity and conviction rather than coercion and control. After a brief review of the literature on leadership, this chapter describes an approach to leadership for general practice, and considers its implications.

Introduction

Writing during the UK general election campaign of 1997, the concept of *primus inter pares* is very much in mind. This concept appears always to have been applied to our prime ministers inaccurately when they hold their office and command their cabinets with obvious authority. Yet 'first among equals' is an epithet that fits. The prime minister has the authority of two mandates – one from the electorate as a member of Parliament, and the other from his parliamentary colleagues as elected leader. In our parliamentary system, these give him or her the authority to lead until either mandate needs to be renewed.

This chapter addresses the theme of leadership in the world of general practice and also in primary care. I do not intend to use general practice and primary care interchangeably. I would like to address general practice first and then widen the debate to primary care. I shall consider general practice, however, on a national scale and primary care at the practice level. In doing so, I am aware that feathers may ruffle at some of the ideas here yet I do so as a great believer in both general practice and primary care, wishing them both well. Still, I may be rushing in where angels fear to tread!

A flat world

General practice is a flat world. Each general practitioner is an independent contractor and each principal is a peer: fully fledged and his or her own boss. There are no bosses in the traditional sense (although some senior partners may do a very good impression of a boss, much to the frustration and annoyance of the other partners).

Leadership is a curious concept in such a world where consensus tends to rule both *de facto* and *de jure*. Yet, leadership is an issue. There is an academic discipline called general practice, and there is the professional activity of general practice also. In the academic world, there are bodies and hierarchies that set and monitor academic standards. University departments monitor standards through examinations. At undergraduate level, courses have to be passed in order for the student to proceed. The university delegates to the academic staff of the various departments authority to speak for the discipline in question. External examiners are also appointed to ensure comparability of standards between institutions. Similar principles are at work at postgraduate level where theses have to be examined, although the emphasis is more on views of external specialists in the field being examined.

Professional practice is not like this. There are no hierarchies. So who speaks for good practice? How are standards set and monitored? How do I know that my children will be treated by a competent GP? Once a doctor is licensed in the UK, he or she can practise without scrutiny until retirement 30 years later. The case for re-accreditation is compelling in as important a discipline as general practice, yet this is not my subject here. Wiser and better qualified opinions than mine have been expressed on this subject, though I have to say that I am heartily in favour.

My subject is leadership – and I want to set out ideas that may make the subject seem less unpalatable in a flat world. I want to show that there are models of leadership that work through positive rather than negative means – through clarity and conviction rather than coercion and control. These models are appropriate for general practice at the local and national levels. There are also 'bosses' who, though they have clear authority, have learned that it is self-defeating to be bossy. These models will work at the local level for primary care.

Models of leadership

The very notion of leadership conjures up images of authority, even domination. Yet the study of leadership soon dispels them. Certainly, there was a time when leadership attributes were investigated. The notion of the commanding presence even gained some brief validity recently when an American commentator observed that, since the arrival of television, the taller of the candidates for the US presidency has always won, with the exception of Jimmy Carter, and there were special reasons for that post Watergate. But 'towering' figures such as Napoleon, Hitler and Gandhi seem to undermine the commanding presence hypothesis, and suggest that there are different styles of leadership.

One key dimension on which leaders differ is their concern for task or process – a dimension that is frequently mentioned in the context of medical care. This matter was researched rather well by Blake and Mouton, who distinguished leaders who were task oriented (they called this 'initiating structure') from those who were more concerned with people (called 'consideration').[1] They found that each style had its obvious strengths but also significant weaknesses. Among the latter, they noticed that those who were high on consideration alone frequently ducked difficult issues and avoided giving challenging feedback. Those high on task orientation alone produced feelings in those around them that threatened job satisfaction and commitment. The research found that it was both possible and most effective to be high on both dimensions.

In psychology, the idea of 'situational leadership' proposed in 1982 by Hersey and Blanchard has gained some credibility.[2] The basic idea is that different styles of leadership are required as the maturity of the followers grows. When maturity or experience is low, a high level of structure is required; as maturity and experience grow, a higher level of social support is needed. When maturity and experience are high, supervision becomes superfluous.

In many ways, these ideas track the emerging clinician's experiences. During medical school, it is the directive teaching process that gives structure to the student's life in medicine. During the registrar period, especially in general practice, the trainer relationship tends to be high on support and lower on structure. As the fully fledged professional emerges, the need for supervision becomes superfluous.

Certainly, there are situations in which leadership is redundant. Kerr and Jermier proposed four substitutes for leadership; the first and most compelling was when the workers were highly skilled or committed.[3] Everyday general practice displays these characteristics. Or does it? That most GPs are highly skilled, there can be little doubt. Yet what is the current state of commitment? There is an increasing loss of morale in GPs that is sad to witness and that is threatening commitment. This is not just in general practice either. Doctors are suffering significant reductions in morale according to countless studies (see *The Times*, 22 April, 1997). Could this suggest that some form of leadership is missing?

Possibly the best recent study of leadership is that provided in 1985 by Warren Bennis and Burt Nanus, who interviewed 90 outstanding leaders from many different walks of life.[4] They interviewed leaders in public service as well as commercial leaders and leaders from the fields of music and sports. Naturally, the leaders differed significantly from each other, but the researchers set out to discover the actions that they all took – the behaviours they shared – in the belief that these similarities would tell them about leadership in gencral. They identified four such shared actions. Described in my words, these are: the creation of a compelling vision; the creation of an aligned community; the creation and maintenance of trust; and the relentless pursuit of improvement. I shall describe each of these actions in a little detail and then consider their possible relevance to the world of general practice.

The creation of vision

Outstanding leaders create focus. They do not dissipate their own or their organisation's energy on what is unimportant. They focus on what is important and draw people towards it by showing its power and desirability. They are obsessed with the outcomes they want to create. Their vision, or dream, is defined so specifically that no one around them is left in any doubt about it. It is a goal that they cannot either relinquish or dilute. It is their driving force, and the values it requires are also the personal values of the leader.

General practice has been like this and the passionate writings of the founders of the Royal College of General Practitioners (RCGP) set out elements of vision in this compelling way. Their *The future general practitioner* report is a good example.[5]

The creation of an aligned community

Outstanding leaders take people with them. They recruit people who share their dream or convert people to it. Those who cannot become aligned with the vision tend to leave as life becomes extremely uncomfortable for them. Their choice is stark – they can modify the vision, live it, or leave.

The means for creating alignment are all loosely concerned with communication rather than compulsion but communication of very different kinds. Personal contact with the leaders leaves everyone very clear about what is important – not just by listening to what they say but by observing what they do. Written communication tends to confirm the vision from letters to journals. The recruitment and appraisal systems similarly embody the vision and values and all who prosper in such an organisation do so by adherence to the vision and values they are pursuing together. People are proud to belong to such organisations.

The alignment of general medical practitioners in this sense is not great. There is no unanimity of view. They have rather sought a broad church in their professional bodies in which tolerance of difference has been the norm. The RCGP could rightly leave it to the General Medical Services Committee to define 'bad' or unacceptable practice. Regrettably, this allowed variations in quality to emerge as succeeding generations considered they had no mandate or special knowledge to define 'better'.

More recently, this is changing for the better. The examiners of the RCGP took on the challenge first, facing the criticism of offended members. The *What sort of doctor?* working parties also proposed criteria for the evaluation of practice and these have formed the basis of other initiatives for judging quality, such as the training practice evaluation visit and methodology, and fellowship by assessment.

The creation and maintenance of trust

People trust outstanding leaders because they are consistent. Their actions, their conversation, their speeches, and their work derive from the same set of values. They have integrity in the strictest sense – all the pieces fit together. The vision and values of the leaders are embodied in their behaviour. They can even be challenged by their subordinates to live in greater conformity with their values if the challenge makes their vision more likely.

Consistency is not to be confused with comfort. Men and women with a burning vision are not necessarily very comfortable to be around. They may even be disliked, but they are trusted. Trust in leaders in general practice is equally important and is likely to be gained and maintained through similar means. Consistency is key.

The relentless pursuit of improvement

Outstanding leaders know their strengths and nurture them. They push to improve themselves and their colleagues are expected to do likewise. They will also accept a level of risk in order to improve their standards. In this way, they accept mistakes as learning opportunities and do not create anxiety about errors. This is not to say that they allow standards ever to drop, merely that their first response is to understand why the error occurred so that some more effective way may be found of avoiding a similar error in the future. They concentrate on success and improvement, rather than failure and blame. In this way they create learning organisations rather than bureaucracies.

This does not mean that they avoid evaluation so as not to offend. They evaluate regularly and enthusiastically so that standards can be raised. There is a challenge for general practice here, and partnerships could lead the way to establishing a norm for formative evaluation and/or appraisal.

Leadership for general practice

Nationally, the Royal Colleges lead in their respective professional disciplines. Regionally, there are the directors of postgraduate medical education. What expectations of their leadership might we legitimately encourage? I believe that we should look for the following four contributions:

1 *Vision*: a statement about the future and our place in it

2 *Mission*: what we must do to turn our vision into reality

3 *Values*: how we must guide our actions

4 *Methods*: the practical manifestation of our vision, mission and values.

Vision, *mission*, and *values* are the most important contributions that leaders make to organisations. They are occasionally considered separately, at other times interchangeably, yet each factor has a unique contribution to make and each one requires the other two. Vision inspires, mission directs, values guide; and each influences the motivation and commitment people feel to the organisations to which they belong. Methods that are consistent with the vision, mission, and values of general practice often require considerable amounts of development time. The RCGP and/or the regional directors have access to appropriate resources to develop them.

Vision

This motivates, inspires and energises. It is not entirely rational – it is a mixture of thinking and feeling. It also need not be expressed in words – it can be a picture or an image. Its function is to show how the future can be better than today. Cathay Pacific Airways' vision is to be found in the first line of its mission statement – called the Cathay Pacific Commitment For The Nineties. It is quite simple: it states – *We will be the airline of the decade,* and goes on to show what they must do in order to bring about this bold ambition.

According to John Kotter, a vision (and mission) needs to be: imaginable, desirable feasible, focused, flexible and communicable.[6] Sir John Harvey-Jones, who led ICI through many of its most successful years, believes a vision should present an attractive and clear view of the future which can be shared. It must motivate, be ambitious and should stretch people to achieve more than they might ever have thought possible. In the 1960s, when Martin Luther King declared that he had a dream – he was sharing his vision with an audience of millions. His dream was of a world in which people would be judged by their character rather than by the colour of their skin. It cost him his life but it brought about change on a massive scale.

Vision in organisations does not need to be so momentous – indeed it rarely can be – but it inspires or it should not be called vision at all. It also focuses on outcomes. When Warren Bennis and Burt Nanus interviewed 90 outstanding leaders while researching their book on leadership, they became impressed by their interviewees and spoke frequently of their 'unparalleled concern with outcome'.[4] They quote an interview with Edwin H Land, the founder of Polaroid, which elegantly demonstrates the preoccupation with outcome and the need to inspire through vision. He stated that:

> … the first thing you naturally do is teach the person to feel that the undertaking is manifestly important and nearly impossible. That draws out the kind of drives that make people strong.

Vision for general practice should be able to inspire as there are such powerful motivators involved. Health and healthcare are powerful potential motivators. The possibility of influencing the health of a practice population and providing well-researched healthcare should be compelling elements of that vision. The trust, respect and affection extended to so many GPs are additional elements. The downside of practice life is not to be underplayed but surely it is more than counterbalanced by the joy. Many people in many professional jobs cannot get close to this sense that their work is worthwhile.

Mission

If vision inspires and shows what could be, mission clarifies and shows how the dream is to be achieved – it tells people what to do in order to turn their dream into reality. It focuses attention and action, turning vision into an obsession. Fuji Film used to have a simple and effective slogan: Kill Kodak! In these two words they focused the attention of all of their employees on the main target of their activity.

In Cathay Pacific's Commitment For The Nineties, their dream of becoming the airline of the decade was to be realised by several specific activities such as putting safety and security first, being totally customer-driven, producing superior financial returns, providing rewarding and enjoyable careers for staff, and so on. The commitment combined *vision* and *mission* into one brief statement.

The British Institute of Management published a survey in 1992 that highlighted the critical role of vision and mission.[7] Since many companies were experiencing rapidly changing environments, they asked their respondents to rate the factors they considered important in creating a new philosophy of management in their companies. By far the most frequently cited was 'clear vision and mission', and 74% rated this item as very important or critical.

Visions and missions have to capture the best the organisation can be, express it succinctly and influence the behaviour of all prominent senior personnel. These are the basic preconditions for the vision and mission to play a part in changing the organisation. Then the mission statement expresses the aspirations to which the organisation is committed, and the rest of the organisation will come to recognise its power.

In general practice, a simple statement of vision would need to be 'unpacked' into the steps that will bring it about (mission). Sadly, it will not usually be possible to draw on empirical research to justify the elements of mission. These come from statements of conviction, determination and logic. They are rhetorically powerful but not empty. They carry the passion and commitment of those who sign up to them.

Values

These guide and support the vision and mission. Here, one may tell the difference between visions and missions that make a difference and those that fail to do so. When effective leaders are fully committed to their vision and mission, their own values and those required to support the vision become one. Bennis and Nanus put it well:[4]

> Leaders acquire and wear their visions like clothes. Accordingly, they seem to enrol themselves (and then others) in the belief of their ideals as attainable, and their behaviour exemplifies the ideals in action.

There are two versions of the values that operate in an organisation – the explicit and the implicit. Explicit values are to be found in formal statements. They are embodied in the rhetoric found in annual reports and formal speeches. They are important and meaningful only when they are found to be true by those who work closely with the organisation.

The *real* values – or at least those that are most widely believed – are the implicit values. These are the values inferred from the behaviour of senior people and that underpin its systems and procedures. They are to be found in the unrehearsed comment, in the stories told in restaurants about the organisation, and in the actions taken in difficult circumstances. When a practice claims to value people but hires and fires them easily, there is little doubt that the rhetoric is false. When a practice claims to value patients but fails to treat them with respect, the same is true. Powerful and effective leaders are intolerant of any significant differences between rhetoric and reality – either in themselves or in others – and act to reconcile the differences swiftly, if at all possible.

Methods

Aspirations or values without methods are deeply frustrating. They become oppressive. This was a lesson that several of us learned most powerfully when teaching about the consultation in general practice. We first used to lecture about the research showing that patient involvement led to greater compliance with medical advice. We then frequently had to deal with objections from the course participants. At first, we would argue the case at length. We learnt not to do this, but rather to ask that we move straight to the part of the course dealing with consulting skills and then revisit the matter. Once the participants learned how relatively easy it is to consult in an involving way, they became more convinced of the need to do so. They had not yet seen any real advantages, they had simply learned that they could do it. Giving them a practical method had freed them up to change their values.

General practitioners do not resist making improvements to their practice, although they sometimes resist change merely for the sake of novelty. They need to be realistic and practical. Using video-recordings of real consultations for teaching only succeeded when the criteria for judging them could be agreed and when practical teaching was offered on how to make such learning work well. The same can be said for computerisation, practice visiting for peer review, and so on. Methods can make change happen quickly. In their absence, new ideas seem like yet more burdens or mere empty rhetoric.

The heart and the periphery

Currently, in the National Health Service, there is considerable doubt and uncertainty. There are changes demanded frequently and an increasing depression about what is being lost. The old values of the NHS conceived by Bevan seem to be fading in face of the increasingly managerial emphasis brought about over the years by Griffiths, Response Allocation Working Party, the purchaser–provider split, fundholding, primary care groups and clinical governance.

However, values need not be threatened by any of these initiatives. Our values are our values. What has changed is that there is now a large number of 'urgent' tasks that are required to obtain funding – many of which are bureaucratic. These do not change what we regard as important, but they can distract us so often that we lose sight of the important, confusing it with that which is required.

Here is an additional leadership challenge – to remind us what is important. It is a part of the creation of vision, mission and values that we identify that which is important and that which is not. This is best achieved by involving people in its creation. Yet, who holds the vision, cares about it and reminds us all of it when we become confused? The answer might be 'every one' but that can so easily mean 'no one'.

As changes are required, there are two kinds: those that are merely additional to the activities that lie at the heart of general practice, and those that are antithetical. There are very few of the latter. The bureaucratic tasks required by fundholding may be arduous but are merely additional. Changing the nature of the doctor–patient relationship from advocate to resource manager may be antithetical but how would we ever know? There appears to be nobody that is authoritative about the matter. Who will take a view? Many people may choose to wade into the argument, but who can claim to know or to speak with authority? Who has the mandate? The RCGP or the regional directors can claim a right to make pronouncements but none has a clear mandate to speak for general practice.

Jennifer King's Chapter 3, however, describes a bold venture to build a consensus in the Oxford Region. Their task is to identify the values and behaviours that lie at the heart of the role of registrar (GP), trainer and course organiser. They hope to become so clear about the core of each role that they can use the statements as touchstones when changes seem to be confusing. They can then embody these ideas in recruitment, appraisal and evaluation criteria. This is leadership in action – the kind to which nobody can object. It is built on consensus, at the heart of general practice, right for the times, and designed to meet a need for clarity.

What of primary care?

Debates about leadership in primary care are even more contentious than those in general practice. Primary care is multidisciplinary and there is resistance to the idea that the leadership of the primary care team should inevitably lie with the GP. The argument is soundly made that the leader may need to be whomsoever is best suited to the role irrespective of discipline, or that leadership could be shared.

I take a very pragmatic stance here. I believe that primary care is made up of practices and that practices have owners. Ownership bestows leadership or the right to appoint leaders. This does not resolve the question at the highest level, since medical ownership is not necessary. Practice teams could own practices, or the local supermarket could own the practice. Indeed, it is becoming increasingly common that a group of owners employ part-time or full-time doctors as well as other allied professions.

This raises the matter of the model of leadership and management that owners might assert. Fortunately, the managerial literature is replete with studies that show that involving, empowering and supportive management produces the best results – even in the most unexpected places. One of the most powerful studies was conducted among sales teams. It showed that the climate the manager created affected powerfully the results the teams produced. When the manager was supportive, challenging, gave recognition, encouraged participation, facilitated self-expression and was clear about what was important, the teams worked harder and produced better results.[8]

Conclusion

Turbulent times call for leadership. The models outlined in this chapter are compatible with the ethos of a caring profession. They could make a powerful and timely contribution to general practice and primary care.

The models of leadership that work best are clear and coherent. They work through clarity and conviction rather than coercion and control. They communicate passionately and inspire commitment. They are well understood, well researched and readily learned. The task is to bring out the best in our colleagues and in ourselves.

Summary

Leadership in general practice is required to enhance standards, advance the discipline and maintain morale. Yet leadership carries inappropriate connotations of control rather than facilitation.

There are many different approaches to leadership and to its study. The ideas of Warren Bennis and Burt Nanus are particularly helpful in this context. Their study of the actions of 90 outstanding leaders pointed to the need for: the creation of a compelling vision, the creation of an aligned community, the creation and maintenance of trust, and the relentless pursuit of improvement.

In general practice, there is a need for leadership. The RCGP and the regional directors of general practice need to be encouraged to make four leadership contributions. They need to create statements about the future and the preferred place of general practice in it. They need to state what needs to be done to turn the vision into reality. They need to identify the values that will guide actions. They also need to devise methods to bring about the vision, mission and values specified.

In this way, leaders will maintain the core of primary care that will be sustained whatever the current initiative from government or challenge posed by our society. They will also discover that principled leadership that mixes challenge and support works most effectively for all those involved.

References

1 Blake R R and Mouton J S (1985) *The managerial grid III.* Gulf, Houston.
A helpful way of thinking about the distinction between task and process in the context of management and leadership.

2 Hersey P and Blanchard K (1982) *Management of organisational behaviour* (4e). Prentice-Hall, Englewood Cliffs.
Describes situational leadership emphasising the context of the follower group's attributes and the leadership responses.

3 Kerr S and Jermier J M (1978) Substitutes for leadership: their meaning and measurement. *Organisational Behaviour and Human Performance,* **22**:375–403.
Suggests four factors that may make a leader's contributions irrelevant: (1) a high

level of knowledge, commitment or experience; (2) job structure; (3) work norms and strong feelings of cohesion; (4) technology.

4 Bennis W and Nanus B (1985) *Leaders: the strategies for taking charge.* Harper and Row, New York.
A truly inspired piece of writing, informative and easy to read. If anyone wants to read just one book on leadership it should be this one.

5 Royal College of General Practitioners (1972) *The future general practitioner.* Report of a working party. British Medical Journal Publications/RCGP, London.
A classic – authoritative and still relevant.

6 Kotter J P (1996) *Leading change.* Harvard Business School Press, Boston.
A lucid and helpful book by an extremely well respected thinker on managerial and leadership issues. Incidentally, he also predicts challenging attributes of the 21st century organisation.

7 Coulson-Thomas C (1992) *Transforming the company.* Kogan Page, London.
A management text that extensively quotes data from the British Institute of Management 1991 surveys.

8 Brown S B and Leigh T W (1996) A new look at psychological climate and its relationship to job involvement, effort and performance. *Journal of Applied Psychology*, **81**:358–68.
An experimental piece in an academic journal. The only article I know that demonstrates the effect of climate on performance and makes good use of the data.

3

Ancient virtues in modern times: values in general practice

Jennifer King

We shall not cease from exploration
And the end of all our exploring
Will be to arrive where we started
And know the place for the first time

T.S. Eliot, *Four Quartets*

Outline

Prompted by the relentless changes in general practice, general practitioner course organisers in Oxford wanted to re-examine their values and professional standards of behaviour. Their aims were twofold: (1) to re-establish some optimism and clarity of purpose among the group; and (2) to produce a document for future vocational training which would guide future recruitment, appraisal and development of GP registrars. This chapter describes the beginning of that process, from the facilitator's viewpoint. It analyses the concepts of values and professional behaviours applied in the general practice context, and offers some generic principles about the process to help other groups undertake a similar exercise.

Background

General practice has undergone unprecedented change in recent years. The range of demands has increased, pulling many general practitioners in different directions. Many GPs have lost sight of what is really important in general practice and have struggled to maintain focus and coherence in their work. As a result, morale is frequently low. The reduction in the numbers of doctors entering general practice, together with the increase in those leaving the profession, is forcing many GPs to reassess what they want from their professional careers and the kind of practice they will be faced with in the future. In the light of all this, the Oxford Region advisers and GP course organisers expressed a need to re-establish what is most essential to general practice. The purpose was to set the scene for future vocational training in general practice, and to focus on the educational and career needs of new GPs. The working document that they planned to produce was intended to guide recruitment, appraisal and professional development of future registrars.

This chapter is an opportunity to describe – as facilitator of this process – some of the insights and lessons from this challenging exercise. At a time when many GP teachers are re-evaluating their role, it is hoped that these insights might prove interesting and helpful to others wishing to tackle similar issues in their own region.

To begin the process and to set it in context, the course organisers began by identifying what they perceived as some of the most important celebrations and frustrations of recent years.

Celebrations and frustrations

There is still much to celebrate in the field of general practice. The change in the out-of-hours arrangements has meant less stress for doctors. Many practices and doctors have embraced the new technologies now available and have used them as an opportunity for innovation. Similarly, fundholding has produced many rewards and benefits, including improved buildings, facilities, staff numbers and better practice organisation and management. The boundaries between doctors and nurses are breaking down. Working patterns are more flexible, with greater scope for women and part-time doctors. People are questioning more openly the value and role of hospital posts for training. The profile of primary care within the National Health Service has increased significantly. In all of this, the doctor–patient relationship has remained key and GPs still enjoy high status within the community and autonomy in their work.

Alongside the celebrations are a number of frustrations which have resulted in low morale and increased job stress for many GPs. The introduction of the 1990 New Contract led to considerable resentment, anger and frustration over what was widely regarded as an inappropriate government imposition. Many felt that it shifted the balance of general practice inappropriately. Largely as a result of this, GPs were expected to do not only more clinical work than before, but also administration, management, negotiation, budgeting and purchasing. Restrictions on time and funds have always been prominent. A severe recruitment crisis has led to increased pressure within the service. Many GPs feel a constant tension between the managerial and administrative demands and those of their patients and between the doctor as patient advocate and as controller of the practice budget. Similar tension persists between service and education demands in vocational training. The growth of information technology and an increasingly consumerist society put much greater demands on the medical profession. Lack of positive feedback is also a problem for doctors in training as well as for established GPs. 'How are we doing?' is not a question often enough addressed. There is currently no well-defined career structure within general practice.

Changes in general practice

So much change has already occurred, with still more to come, that it helps to highlight the most important areas of change – past and imminent – and to consider some possible implications for future general practice and vocational training.

Many of the recent changes are described in (and often a result of) the 1996 Department of Health White Paper, *Primary care: the future – choice and opportunity*.[1] In general, societal changes have brought about increased patient expectations, greater multiracial needs, increased demands in the profession for better balance between personal and professional life. In addition, there is growing interdependence between primary and secondary care, as well as changing boundaries between the roles of the GP and other primary care professionals – especially with the expansion of the nurse's role. Overall, the organisation of primary healthcare is becoming more team-based. There is also a significant move towards evidence-based medicine. Information technology brings new challenges in sharing and evaluating information, balancing community needs and choices for patients.

Imminent changes can be separated into those likely to affect general practice and those affecting vocational training and education. In general practice, the increased responsibilities being devolved to nurses and other primary care professionals will result in the service becoming more uniform. We are already starting to see the emergence of 'one-stop shops'; surgeries and pharmacists being established in supermarkets and railway stations; health facilities, such as a gym, on the surgery premises. Working arrangements will need to become more flexible to take account of increasing numbers of part-time doctors. Future generations of GPs may not want to stay in general practice for their whole working life, perhaps preferring mixed careers and more career development opportunities. The change in the out-of-hours arrangements was a direct reflection of GPs' need for a more acceptable balance between personal and professional life.

Vocational training, for the first time since its introduction in the early 1970s, is seeing a dissolution of the rigid pattern of twelve months in general practice and two years in hospital. The new Vocational Training Scheme regulations from the Department of Health are becoming much more flexible and, where funding allows, permit training in general practice to be extended to eighteen months. The introduction of summative assessment appears to have raised the standards of training in some practices, but it will be a while before the proper effects have been evaluated. Trainers and course organisers will need to review the traditional methods of learning and teaching, with more emphasis on self-directed, problem-based and experiential learning in their registrars. Training and curricular needs will require more negotiation. More collaboration will be required with other disciplines.

The recent Department of Health White Paper (1998), *The NHS: modern, dependable*, proposes some significant changes to the way primary care is structured.[2] There is the proposed formation first, of primary care trusts and second, of primary care groups. The latter will have considerable implications for how GPs and practices work together – for how they build and pursue a common vision and goals, for leadership within the group and for managing and working as part of a very large group.

Implications of change

The full implications of some of these changes have yet to be felt. At such times, especially after prolonged or momentous change, those affected need to regain some equilibrium – to view the past in perspective, with all its strengths as well as frustrations, and to look to the future with some clarity, optimism and sense of purpose. It is important to know what to retain and what to replace. One typical response at such times is to focus unerringly on reorganising structures and systems – a new system of financial accounting, for example; a new method of clinical audit; new staff reporting structures. There is a growing recognition that this approach overlooks the people involved and their feelings about change. Kenneth Clarke's reorganisation of the health service in the late 1980s no doubt seemed a logical way to tackle inefficiencies and cut costs – but it was criticised for failing to take account of the fundamental professional *values* of general practice. Many GPs felt forced into a way of working that sharply conflicted with their values – in particular their need for autonomy.

The prevailing climate of emotional distress in many parts of the health service derives in part from people feeling undervalued. Many say that the values that brought them into the service originally are being eroded by increasing workload and pressure to reconcile the priorities of management with those of patient care. General practitioners have reacted in part by re-rooting themselves in family values and by more emphasis on personal needs.

Building a vision

> The ability to manage continuity and change is closely linked to the ability to develop a vision. Vision provides guidance about what core to preserve and what future to stimulate progress toward.[3]

Recent experience of working with several general practices shows clearly that those who have thrived most in the face of change are those who have a clear vision that all staff in the practice can support. Those who have floundered have invariably lacked this vision, which was due in turn to an absence of leadership. Practices which are strong internally can better withstand external uncertainty. A yachting analogy is relevant – when the tides and currents are constantly changing and unpredictable, the yacht can remain on course provided it knows the direction in which it is headed. A strong helmsman and a sturdy crew will keep the course steady.

The challenge for the Oxford Region general practitioner course organisers was to set their course by identifying their vision of the future. Vision has two key components: *purpose* and *values.* For example, Hewlett Packard's purpose is not to make electronic equipment but to make technical contributions to improve people's lives. Walt Disney's purpose is not to make cartoons but to make people happy. Change causes people to re-examine their purpose and *raison d'être.* Calman described the purpose of medicine as being 'to serve the community by continually improving health, healthcare and quality of life for the individual and the population …'[4] Change stimulated the Oxford course organisers to reflect on the purpose of their role, to ensure that it would reflect changing needs and help them to guide future GP registrars.

Discussing values and purpose is challenging because they are at the heart of what matters to us most. When other things around us are in constant flux it helps to remember our most passionate beliefs. People may find these hard to express: (1) such beliefs may be absent; (2) they may be subconscious; (3) they may be conscious but unexpressed; (4) they may be expressed but hard to prioritise. It helps to understand that values are not what you should believe but what you do believe. They are not created but discovered. Most importantly – they are discovered through the heart not the head – they are what we feel rather than what we think. Goleman's book *Emotional intelligence*[5] reminds us of the importance of bringing more emotion to our decisions and actions and not relying solely on intellect which – as Einstein said – 'has powerful muscles but no personality'. Roger Neighbour's book *The inner consultation* talks about using intuition – a concept highly relevant to identifying values.[6]

Values and behaviours

How do values come alive? How does a profession or organisation ensure that its values are upheld? What kind of behaviour is expected? For example, consider the finest GP trainer you have ever encountered. What made this trainer's behaviour exceptional? How did it differ from the behaviour of a trainer that you might describe as 'average'? Being able to distinguish the best from the rest helps to raise people's sights and identify a set of professional behaviours which, together with values, comprise a standard of excellence. The jargon in this area is often confusing – management literature increasingly refers to these behaviours as 'competencies'. This can be misleading when you consider that the dictionary defines competency as 'sufficient' or 'adequate'. Many understand 'competency' to mean simply a skill or ability. Indeed, so frequent is the confusion generated by the term 'competency' that – while accepting that it may be commonly used – it is more helpful to the current discussion simply to use the term 'behaviour'. This should be qualified by saying that we mean behaviour which distinguishes the exceptional from the average. So, to recap:

- *Values* are about what is most important
- *Behaviours* in this context are characteristic of the best practitioners, and are consistent with values
- *Skills, knowledge,* and *attitudes* are the building blocks of behaviour and help to account for the superior performance.

Identifying values

There have been several important publications embodying the values of the medical profession and of general practice in particular.

These have provided an invaluable starting point from which to reappraise values for current and future general practice and its teaching. They include the General Medical Council (GMC) guidelines,[7] *What sort of doctor?*,[8] *Priority objectives for general practice vocational training*,[9] *The future general practitioner: learning and teaching*,[10] and Calman's 1994 article, 'The profession of medicine'.[4]

The GMC guidelines are fundamentally important. They identify a number of behaviours considered essential for all doctors. For example, the doctor must:

- treat every patient politely and considerately
- respect every patient's dignity and privacy
- listen to patients and respect their views
- give patients information in a way they can understand
- respect the rights of patients to be fully involved in decisions about their care
- be honest and trustworthy
- respect and protect confidential information
- work with colleagues that best serve patients' interests.

The *Priority objectives*, under the heading of 'professional values', describes the personal attitudes and values regarded as fundamental to the good general practitioner. Examples are: awareness of own values, beliefs and attitudes; tolerance, respect and flexibility; willingness to give and receive criticism, and awareness of factors that influence the relationships between personal and professional life.

Similarly, *The future general practitioner* provides a detailed account of educational objectives which itself incorporates a number of values, such as self-criticism, as being essential for a good teacher. Calman, in his paper 'The profession of medicine', talks about commitment and compassion as being very important to a doctor's work and goes on to list several 'key values expected of doctors': these include (among others) a high standard of ethics, continuing professional development, the ability to work in a team, concern with clinical standards and ability to communicate.

When reviewing these publications it is evident that the values of the GP have altered little in the last 12–15 years – with two exceptions. The first is a resurgence of family values. The young generation of doctors are now much more determined to seek a balance between their personal and working lives and are no longer prepared always to put their patients before themselves or their families. The second emerging value is working as part of a team. A far higher percentage of care is now given by non-doctors. The contribution of other team members to providing high quality care is now recognised and more highly valued.

The challenges

Revisiting these publications posed a number of fundamental challenges. The first was to decide how things have changed since these earlier documents were written. The very multiplicity of the values expressed is confusing – hence the need to decide what to preserve for the future and to ensure that the current values reflected changing times.

The second challenge was how to maintain core values in the light of the current recruitment crisis in general practice. Given the diminishing quality and quantity of new recruits to the profession, are values an unaffordable luxury? The debate raised two further questions: 'When recruiting, how can you tell whether a potential GP registrar shares our values?' and 'Can we train new doctors to hold these values?'. Collins and Porras' article is helpful here, suggesting the following:[3]

> A clear and well-articulated ideology attracts people whose personal values are compatible with (the company's) core values; conversely it repels those whose personal values are incompatible. You cannot impose core values on people. How do we get people to share our core ideology? You don't. You can't. Instead, find people who are pre-disposed to share your core values – attract and retain those people.

A third challenge was how to access values by using feelings rather than intellectual analysis. Asking people to think of the finest example of, say, general practice teaching, and what *felt good* about it is often a helpful way to begin. Asking people to think about what matters most, who is most important to them and why, what areas of their life or work they would refuse to compromise on are all questions which start the process of identifying values.

Much effort has been spent in medicine trying to produce value statements. It is tempting to try to produce a definitive form of words and a perfect statement – which often results in a weak dilution of the original essence. In this case, it was agreed that the important aim was to focus on distilling that essence in a way that could later be expressed in many different ways.

The following was the initial statement of values for general practice, as expressed by the Oxford Region GP Course Organiser group. It is not a final or definitive statement and has since continued to be debated and refined. The great strengths of the following lines are that they manage to capture most of what is still core to general practice as well as reflecting changes in society and the profession:

> A general practitioner is an enthusiastic generalist whose prime concern is to care for his/her patients and the communities in which they live. In his/her relationships with patients the good general practitioner is warm, open, deals with patients individually and holistically and especially values the one-to-one relationship with them. S/he maintains a high standard of clinical skills and knowledge, using the best evidence available. S/he is committed to life-long learning and professional development and works as part of a team. S/he balances personal and professional commitments with flexibility and develops ways to handle pressure whilst remaining positive. S/he retains the highest standards of personal integrity.

Identifying key behaviours

So far the focus has been on values in general practice. These values (as expressed above) are the basis for identifying particular key areas of behaviour (i.e. those that distinguish the best from the rest). Some of the behaviours to which a GP trainer should aspire, for example, may be different from essential behaviours for a GP registrar or a GP course organiser. In order to clarify the standards expected of each group, a number of different 'sets' of behaviours needed to be identified. They would all, however, be based on common values.

The *Priority objectives* is an invaluable starting point, identifying four key areas of behaviour in which the GP needs to be competent. These include patient care, communication, organisation, personal and professional growth. The question is: how far do these still apply and how far will they continue to apply in the future? Will they change completely or just assume a different emphasis? Do they adequately reflect the changes within general practice? For example, what about changing professional boundaries; information technology; audit and quality improvement; evidence-based medicine; community-based care; changing from generalist to specialist role, etc.? What are the key behaviours that will be required for these changes? It was already clear, having reviewed the recent changes in general practice, that the list would need to be expanded to include areas such as patient-centred care, balance of personal and professional life, and teamwork. Work continues in Oxford to refine this list in this Region and to provide some specific examples to clarify understanding of the standards expected in each area of behaviour.

As well as essential areas in which all GPs will be involved, there are several optional areas involving only some GPs. These would include clinical areas such as minor surgery; certain aspects of chronic disease management; a variety of management issues – budgets, negotiating, employment contracts; and other issues like running one-stop health shops, supermarket surgeries. High standards must be maintained in these areas, and further work is needed to identify the required professional behaviours that will distinguish the best from the rest in all these activities.

GP registrars

The future general practitioner provides a useful starting point in identifying the competencies of the best GP registrar. It analyses in detail what the GP trainee (now registrar) should have learned by the end of the period of training. Many of the aims are still relevant, although the emphasis may have changed, along with the changing needs of society and the patient. These changes – as mentioned at the start of this chapter – have implications for the recruitment of GP registrars to vocational training, and for the way they learn and develop during training. For example, the changing balance between hospital and GP education; the move towards modular education; the push towards more active rather than passive learning – these require teamworking; self-directed learning and self-development;

dealing with uncertainty. Increasingly, it will be these behaviours that will be expected of the future GP registrar.

GP trainers

> To be trained is to have arrived; to be educated is to continue to travel.[4]

What is to be the role of the future GP trainer? Once again, the *Priority objectives* provides some answers, many of which still apply currently, for example:

- Trainers must be clear what objectives they are attempting to teach
- Learning should be exploited to the full
- Trainers must make adequate initial and subsequent assessments of their trainees (which includes changing the emphasis of learning from one trainee to another according to need).

The changes likely to affect future vocational training clearly imply that the above objectives will be necessary but by no means sufficient for the future. The Oxford Region GP Course Organiser group identified a number of behaviours which they considered essential for future trainers – including motivating through feedback, promoting self-directed learning, being willing to experiment with new methods of teaching, being able to adapt to the changing needs of GP registrars, and several aspects of leadership. Further work is now required to develop a stronger educational focus to these areas and ultimately to decide whether the trainer is – as Calman challenges – a trainer or an educator. Meeting this challenge will require a broad vision and some very clear values for teaching.

GP course organisers

Identifying ideal behaviours for course organisers was, as for trainers, entirely dependent on being able to anticipate what will happen to future vocational training. It seems likely, for example, that schemes will become much more complex; that traditional boundaries between the course organiser and GP tutor may become less distinct; and that the profile of GP education will need continually to be raised with appropriate incentives to attract attendance.

All of these pose considerable challenges to the course organiser. These changes imply that key behaviours must include teamworking, networking and resource investigation; managing change, learner-centred teaching and working with and within groups.

Observations on the process

The process of identifying values and behaviours produced some fascinating lessons and insights. They are generic and do not pertain to any particular group or profession. Any group undertaking a process of this complexity is likely at some stage to experience some of the feelings, dilemmas and challenges that are described here. To keep the focus positive and forward looking, the dilemmas are expressed as a series of recommendations which may serve as a guide to others undertaking a similar exercise:

- *Make all agendas overt* and ensure that everyone is working to the same one
- *Ensure that everyone feels some ownership* of what is produced. Balance the need for collective ownership versus the impracticality of making decisions by committee. This is crucial to the effectiveness of the process. If each member of the group is involved in every stage, progress will be slow and cumbersome and people will start to lose interest. The best solution is to *establish a 'Mars group'* whom others trust to take the process further forward. This is based on the notion that if a small group were to be sent to Mars to promulgate this process, they should consist of those who most clearly understand and best embody the ideas involved. Members of the Mars group are appointed according to these criteria
- *Revisit the purpose and expectations of the exercise when the group hits an inevitable low point.* When people feel their values are being challenged or exposed they lose a sense of purpose and direction. Re-establish a common understanding about what we are trying to do, how we want to do it, and who will take it forward. *Check the following:*
  - Purpose – what do we want this exercise to do for us?

- How do we want the process to work?
- What kind of product or outcome do we want?

- *Balance comprehensiveness with coherence.* There is a tendency to want to include everything when listing key behaviours or values. If too many values are included they are probably not really 'core'. The problem with being too comprehensive is that there is a loss of coherence and focus – both of which are essential to this kind of exercise
- *Engage feelings and intuition* as well as intellect and recognise when and how to achieve the appropriate balance. Revisit people's feelings at various points in the process especially when conflict surfaces
- *Recognise and manage the tension between those who thrive on reflection and debate and those who are more task orientated.* There is tremendous value in debate and reflection and time should be allowed for this. But others will need to see something tangible in order to maintain their commitment. Both needs should be catered for
- *Maintain a balance between process and task.* This is where it helps to have two facilitators (preferably one external and one internal). One can keep the task on track while the other monitors process
- *View conflict as positive rather than negative and help it work for the group.* Recognise that forced consensus is not ultimately productive. No conflict may mean apathy
- *Stay focused as well as positive* (well-placed humour helps!). Negative emotion causes stress and blocks creative thinking and communication.

A final salutary reminder comes from a recent article by Jane MacNaughton:[11]

> … Medicine is above all a practical job with a knowledge base that must be acquired and sustained. There has been an outbreak of 'core values' statements from medical schools as they attempt to redefine the end product of the educational process … let's not forget the medicine.

Conclusions

Having recently reread *The future general practitioner*, one of the Oxford GP course organisers offered a particularly helpful insight: 'Part of the honesty of teaching and training perhaps is also to realise that we are only relearning in our teaching what the past masters had known for many centuries'. A similar view was expressed at a 1994 British Medical Association conference on core values for the medical profession: 'The profession's values are really "ancient virtues distilled over time" but need to be made relevant to modern society'.[12] This indeed will be the challenge.

Summary

- Change in general practice has produced cause for celebration and frustration. The overall effect has been the re-emergence of family values and greater emphasis on personal development.
- Practices which have thrived on change have had a clear vision. Two key components of vision are *values* and *purpose.*
- Values are often difficult to express – they are what *does* matter most, not what *should* matter most. They come from the heart, not from intellectual analysis.
- A profession upholds its values through a series of key behaviours. These are not just any behaviours that all GPs are expected to show – but those which distinguish 'the best from the rest'. Combined with values, these behaviours comprise standards for excellence.
- Some values in general practice have changed in the last 15 years. The context has changed, however, with more emphasis on family values and teamworking.
- The process yielded lessons about ownership of ideas in a large group, maintaining focus and coherence in a potentially 'woolly' exercise, managing tensions between achieving the task and allowing space for reflection and how to access and express values that help build vision.

Acknowledgements

I am indebted to the following: Dr John Hasler for initiating and funding this work in the Oxford Region; Dr David Pendleton for helping to develop many of the ideas; Dr John Horder for his valuable comments on the original draft; Dr Penny Aeberhard for her insights and correspondence; and the Oxford Region GP Course Organiser group of 1997 led by Dr Neil Johnson, for their collective wisdom; and finally Dr Philippa Moreton for her encouragement and editing.

References

1 Department of Health (1996) *Primary care: the future – choice and opportunity*. HMSO, London.

2 Department of Health (1997) *The NHS: modern, dependable*. HMSO, London. These two White Papers, particularly the 1997 document, have major implications for primary healthcare. The introduction to this chapter is based on some of the implications of these two documents.

3 Collins J C and Porras J I (1996) Building your company's vision. *Harvard Business Review*, Sept–Oct:65–74.
This paper was written in a leading management journal but provides a valuable model for any team or organisation building a vision. It explains the key components of vision and helps clarify exactly what is meant by 'core values' and how to access them.

4 Calman K (1994) The profession of medicine. *British Medical Journal*, **309**: 1140–3.
Calman examines the purpose of medicine and its basic values. He gives a particularly clear exposition of key values in addressing the question 'What do doctors need?' and encourages fuller debate in this area. This is a feet-on-the-ground article with great clarity of thought.

5 Goleman D (1995) *Emotional intelligence*. Bloomsbury, London.
An enlightening account of the role of emotions – and the importance of bringing greater emotional intelligence into our lives. The author uses some fascinating medical science as well as many psychological case examples to support his arguments.

In the wake of all the changes in general practice, the ideas in the following publications remain far-sighted, at times inspirational, and still highly relevant. It is context rather than content that has changed. Many of the ideas in these books still apply today, and thus provided a valuable benchmark for the process described in this chapter.

6 Neighbour R (1987) *The inner consultation.* MTP, Lancaster.

7 General Medical Council (1995) *Duties of a doctor.* GMC, London.

8 Royal College of General Practitioners (1985) *What sort of doctor?* Report from General Practice 23. RCGP, London.

9 Oxford Region Course Organisers Group and Regional Advisers Group (1988) *Priority objectives for general practice vocational training* (2e). RCGP, London.

10 Royal College of General Practitioners (1972) *The future general practitioner.* Report of a working party. British Medical Journal Publications/RCGP, London.

11 MacNaughton J (1997) Medicine and the arts: let's not forget the medicine. *British Journal of General Practice*, **48**:952–3.
This article is a timely reminder that the role of the general practitioner is in danger of becoming 'so diffuse as to be meaningless, and the task of designing education for such a role becomes impossible'. The author cautions against losing focus on the central role of the doctor – 'by all means … make our health centres more … attractive, but if we lose the role of delivering *medical* care to our patients then the profession will truly have lost its way'.

12 British Medical Association (1994) *Core values for the medical profession in the 21st century.* Conference report. BMA, London.
This report looks more broadly at medicine rather than just at general practice. It resembles more the first stages of this debate rather than providing a definitive and focused statement of core values. It provides a useful analysis of the different aspects of commitment and the attributes expected of the committed doctor.

4

The development of practice management

Lynne Hobden-Clarke

Outline

This chapter is based on personal experience and observations on the development of practice management. It reviews the way the role of the practice manager has expanded, explores the benefits that strong management can bring to a practice and the ways in which the role continues to evolve.

Introduction

> Hello, I'm from the RCGP and we've heard a rumour that you were a personnel manager for Marks & Spencer and left them to become a practice manager. We can't believe it's true, so I'm 'phoning to check.

This telephone conversation took place in August 1985, approximately two weeks after I had joined a practice in Gerrards Cross. It highlights just how far management in general practice has progressed since the mid 1980s and, instead of being a curiosity, a practice manager with a commercial or business background has become an accepted norm, indeed, a necessity.

The advent of practice management

In the early 1980s, there was a view gathering momentum that general practitioners had a full clinical workload and were beginning to accept that they had neither the skills nor the time to undertake a managerial role. At this point, practice managers were appointed, but primarily as administrators to shoulder the responsibility of finance and paperwork. Most usually they were internal appointments; often a senior receptionist or secretary was promoted and given the title of 'practice manager'. For these reasons the practice manager in 1985 was an almost exclusively female role. In many cases, the range of duties did not really change; many were allocated the task of monitoring practice finance but not given access to partnership profits, and they continued to follow the partners' instructions. In other words, the original managers often did not have a place in the decision-making process of the practice. Obviously, this suited some practice managers in having a grander title, a salary increase and a restricted accountability. Their main function was to carry out the wishes of the partners without challenge or comment.

The role of a practice manager: 1985

> On my first day at Calcot Medical Centre one of the partners advised me that I could make the job as large or as small as I wished. If I wanted to raise the profile of management, the opportunity was there to be taken.

This type of comment is typical of those partners who are prepared to be managed. Those who are prepared to review and justify their actions; who do not resent a non-clinician making informed comment about the practicalities involved in the delivery of primary care; who are willing to be part of and to pool the resources of the whole team and who accept that their expertise is in a specific field. The willingness to give a manager permission to manage distinguishes a forward-looking practice from a complacent one. It is also the biggest single influence on a manager's effectiveness.

Yet, in 1985, the role was largely administrative and centred around organisational issues. There was time to redesign noticeboards and the practice manager had traditionally looked after all the plants in the building. The bulk of time was spent monitoring item of service claim forms sent to the Family Practitioner Committee and checking the correct remuneration was received. There were self-imposed projects, for example, to develop a handbook containing all the terms and conditions of employment, agree job descriptions and introduce an effective appraisal system for the ancillary staff. There was very little training available, except for reception staff, and no common standard or expectation to guide a new manager.

'Neither fish, fowl nor good red meat'

Part of the complexity of the manager's role revolves around their place within the hierarchy and reporting structure of the practice. The manager's responsibilities shift considerably, as does the professional relationship with the partners and other members of the team.

Employee

A practice manager is an employee of the partnership and their position is the same as any other member of staff with regard to their legal status and employment rights.

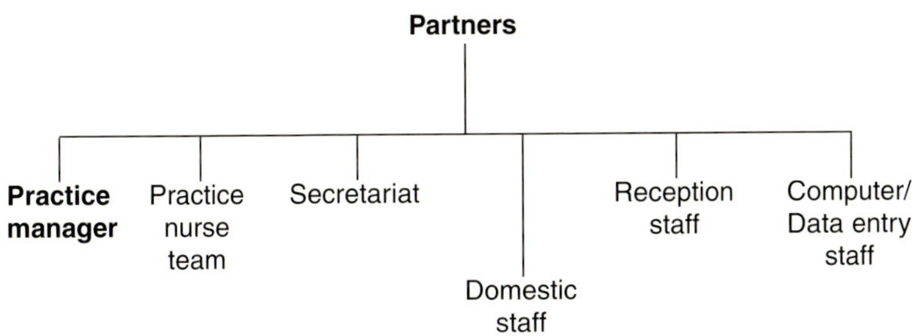

Decision-making

A manager should have a clear place in the decision-making process and then communicate and implement policy decisions. At this point, the manager is on a par with the partners in terms of providing information and as an interface between the partners and the rest of the team.

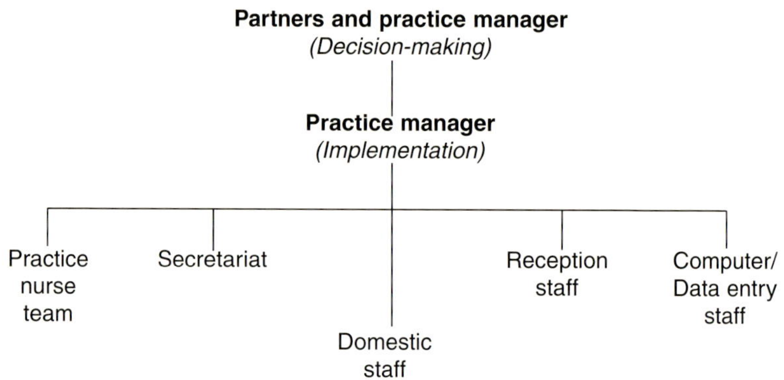

Routine organisation

Once the policy decisions have been agreed and implemented the practice manager becomes responsible for their maintenance, which may include reminding a partner who deviates from the desired norm. The most common example is the equitable distribution of home visits and 'extras', where the practice manager is the final arbiter. In these cases the partners are, in effect, working for the manager.

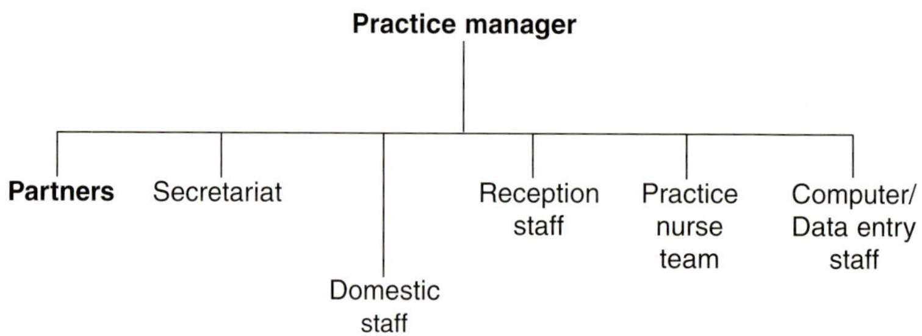

This shifting status can create difficulties, especially if the practice manager is inexperienced and lacks confidence. However, it can also be an enormous strength. The objectivity afforded by such a flexible position can enhance the quality of decisions made because they will be unhindered by bias.

The 1990 New Contract

The 1990 New Contract probably had the greatest impact on general practitioners who were undecided about the merits of practice management and those who felt that delegation was unnecessary. The Contract imposed a number of financial changes by reducing basic allowances and introducing other methods to generate the perceived 'lost' income. The guidelines needed to be fully understood, organisational systems introduced and income maximised. The traditional 'administrator' needed to learn more entrepreneurial and personnel skills. If they were unwilling or lacking in capability the only option was to recruit a manager from a business environment. This spilled over into other areas of the practice when partners realised that to take full advantage of the opportunities offered in the New Contract, they had to delegate. The other group whose numbers increased dramatically during this period were the practice nurses. From this time onwards the place for management in general practice was clearly established.

Fundholding

1991 saw the introduction of fundholding, a very radical concept that introduced a purchaser/provider split within the National Health Service. Those practices who opted to take responsibility for their own budget for practice staff, drugs and appliances and to purchase a restricted range of patient services had to fulfil certain criteria, one of which was the managerial competence and capability of the senior team. Practices found several ways to tackle this issue

– a newly recruited fund manager with finance and business skills, the existing practice manager extending the role to encompass fund management, a partner sharing budgetary responsibility with the manager, or a partner taking full control. Whatever option was chosen, the outcome was the same; the quality of practice management came under close scrutiny. It also brought another dimension into practices which had a practice manager and a fund manager – who was in charge of what? For the majority of duties the division of accountability was clear, except for the staffing budget. Here, both parties had to work in unison, one from a budgetary viewpoint and the other from an operational one. The level of remuneration was another potential stumbling block, especially when fund managers were offered competitive salaries to attract them from other employment.

The role of the practice manager: 1995

The preceding ten years had seen a dramatic change in attitude towards practice managers, both within general practice and from other related bodies. The administrative portion of the role had diminished and the management function enhanced. Common sense had prevailed and managers were being used more appropriately, repetitive tasks were delegated more readily and partnerships were actively seeking good value from the most expensive member of the ancillary staff. This facilitated access to areas that had previously been taboo, for example, strategic planning and the future direction of primary care.

In reality, a manager works for each partner as an individual as well as the partnership as a whole. To speed up routine decision-making (i.e. a small matter that needs the approval of the partners but is too minor to justify waiting for the next practice meeting), many partnerships work on an executive partner system. This allows the practice manager to consult one person for each aspect of practice management (e.g. finance, staffing, audit and the practice nurse team). It also has an added value to the partner concerned as they can use it as an educational opportunity to work with a manager in research, consultation with the team and subsequent implementation of change.

By 1995, practice managers expected to be involved in every area of general practice and had a valuable contribution to make. A suitable aim of the role could be:

> To be responsible for the efficient, effective and safe, administrative and financial management of the practice; to ensure the well-being of patients, doctors and staff and the successful, smooth running of the practice.

The practice manager's duties can be defined under the following headings of responsibility, although many of the specific tasks could, of course, be delegated.

Partnership secretary

This encompasses everything to do with business meetings, their organisation, attendance, minutes and follow-up. Instead of being led by the partnership, a competent manager will be adding items to business meeting agendas and ensuring that ongoing issues are not forgotten; the production of regular reports, cost–benefit analyses for innovations, the partnership agreement, liaison with the practice accountant or any other professional consultant and all confidential partnership matters (e.g. cash withdrawals).

The partners

The practice manager acts primarily as an adviser in the decision-making process and an implementer of policy decisions. He or she has a role as a facilitator for clinical issues, for example, ensuring audit meetings are arranged or an involvement in the out-of-hours rota. It is also the duty of the manager to take the maximum administrative burden from the GPs to allow them to pursue their clinical excellence. In training practices this duty extends to GP registrars who require tutorials and ongoing discussions about managerial topics. In an emotionally mature practice, the manager often assumes the personnel role to the partners, caring for them as people and not simply viewing them dispassionately as employers. This last point is crucial when the partnership is facing a major decision and there are opposing views that may result in conflict. The listening and mediating role is essential in these circumstances.

The staff

The safe recruitment, retention and dismissal of staff requires a working knowledge of current legislation, not only employment but also health and safety. It involves staff contracts, job descriptions, performance reviews, maintaining a level of staffing appropriate to the workload and within a given budget. Staff are a practice's most valuable resource and the team should be developed through training, opportunity and encouragement to achieve their full potential. The practice manager is responsible for maintaining open channels of communication via staff meetings and upholding standards of discipline and codes of conduct.

The patients

The practice manager's contact with patients need not be restricted to dealing with complaints, it should be a much more proactive role. We rarely view the practice from a patient's point of view; for example, telephoning the appointments telephone number to see how we are greeted or how long it takes for the telephone to be answered. Many practices have a patients' charter, but this needs to be audited and monitored if it is to have a benefit to the patients or the practice. Those partnerships who have a patient participation group often appoint the practice manager as the liaison person, and use the group to evaluate potential patient services.

General administration

The bulk of the administrative workload revolves around the health authority and fee or allowance earning claims. In-house paperwork includes written guidance or protocols for all systems, insurance policies, computer and data management. The manager is also responsible for the maintenance of the premises, gardens, car parks, hygiene standards and the security of buildings and personnel. Latterly, this may have included purchasing mobile telephones, organising modem links along with the more mundane ordering of supplies for stationery and practice consumables. This has been the traditional role for a practice manager in general practice.

Finance

Although a practice manager does not need to be an accountant, a thorough knowledge of the *Red Book* and financial principles is essential. The practice accountant will produce audited accounts at the end of each financial year, but in many ways the information arrives too late to be useful. It is much more effective if the manager can maintain quarterly records of income and expenditure and compare them to previously agreed targets and the same quarter in previous years. This will facilitate adjustments during the year and alert the partners to potential shortfalls or surpluses. The manager is also responsible for administering all the salaries within a practice and therefore needs to understand Inland Revenue and National Insurance obligations.

Strategic planning

Now that the production of an annual business plan is required by each health authority, every practice has to agree its aims and objectives for the following financial year. These must include costings when an initiative is to be considered for development money funding. However, real strategic planning is more about attitude than an enforced annual document. It relates to a partnership's ability to view each change as an opportunity to move closer to a longer term ambition. It allows for full and frank discussion, a shared vision and decisions taken as a team based on evidence. The practice manager's role here is invaluable; by keeping up to date with White Papers, Executive Letters and general information they can ensure that a practice is constantly planning and evaluating.

Public relations

Nationally, the social culture reflects a growth in consumerism. Every practice needs a particular number of patients to remain financially viable and the onus is on the practice to attract new patients and retain existing ones. Every person who visits a practice, be they patient or visitor, will formulate an opinion of the practice from what they see and hear. The protection and enhancement of a practice's reputation is properly part of the practice manager's remit. It is reinforced in a number of ways, the most powerful being the personal conduct and behaviour of the manager and partners. There are occasional social functions to organise as well as meetings to which external organisations are invited, and it is the attention to detail at such events that communicates a sense of pride to those who attend.

Confidential matters

There are certain situations that demand the practice manager's personal attention, and these often involve the partners. It may be a formal complaint when the partner concerned needs emotional support and reassurance, as well as a totally confidential wordprocessor.

In summary, a manager in the 1990s needs the same range of skills as any small business owner or the managing director of a medium-sized business. Interestingly, currently there are far more men successfully applying for practice manager vacancies.

The benefits of good management

Good management is invisible – it means being constantly proactive to avoid crises and creating a working environment that recognises the individual's contribution to attain the organisation's goals.

There are some obvious and measurable benefits of competent management, for example, in improving the profitability of the practice or extending the range of patient services. However, many of the advantages are unquantifiable in statistical terms and relate to morale and quality. The greatest influence has probably been on the development of the team. The essential aspects of employment, like contracts and job descriptions, are definite tasks which have legal implications. The real work of management begins when staff are employed and working (*see* Box 4.1).

Box 4.1: Optimal team management

Practice aim
To deliver high quality primary care that is readily accessible and available to all patients

Practice manager
To maintain a cost-effective level of staffing, appropriately trained and equipped, to support the doctors in their clinical activities

Practice nurses
To support the doctors in health promotion activities and the monitoring of chronic disease

Reception team
To make access to a doctor or nurse available, based upon the patient's view of the urgency

Administration
To put the needs of the patients before the needs of bureaucracy

Team building

Setting objectives

Without a common task there is no need for a team, so the first principle of motivating a team is to identify the overall objectives of the organisation. There are a number of ways to do this, for example, a series of partnership and staff meetings, but in the past few years we have seen the introduction of 'away days'. This is simply a term that describes a meeting away from the practice that many, or all, of the team attend. It is facilitated by an appropriately skilled person who will 'manage' the day, design a suitable programme and chair the discussions. The important point is that the day, and any decisions, belongs to the practice team and the facilitator has no place in influencing decisions or judging them. Many partnerships use an away day to agree mission statements and cascade these into specific objectives for each group.

The same principle can be applied to any project or review that the practice deems important enough to involve the whole team. Some practices have had several away days and worked through from mission statements and objectives to new initiatives, for example, to become a training practice, or complete reviews of their patient services. The benefits are unlimited. Irrespective of the topic, the most important is recognition for all staff that their views will be welcomed and taken seriously. This alone will strengthen the team by setting aside undisturbed time to discuss an issue thoroughly and fostering a feeling of ownership for any subsequent outcomes, hence increasing the chances of success. The spin-offs are the opportunities to talk to staff with whom managers do not have daily contact, a general feeling of getting to know everyone better, and viewing issues from all perspectives.

Away days have achieved another, probably unexpected, goal. They have raised the awareness and understanding of team development, team functions and motivational methods. It is quite normal to have a discussion with a manager about Belbin scores, Maslow's hierarchy of human needs and Tuckman's 'forming, storming, norming and performing' theory. When reviewing business plans and the future direction of the practice, techniques such as SWOT (strengths, weaknesses, opportunities and threats) and PESTLE (political, economic, social, technological, legal and ecological) analyses are widely used, the former to look parochially at a practice, the latter to look at the trends in the world and environment around us. These have been standard texts and methods in industry and commerce for many years, and their introduction into general practice marks the growing level of management sophistication and professionalism.

Appraisal

Away days are normally an annual or biannual event, so what happens in between? The answer is the everyday relationships between members of the team, how each individual is developed and how standards are introduced and maintained. The technique designed to allow this type of ongoing process is appraisal and the majority of practices have some form of performance review. It is the personnel parallel of clinical audit. The word 'appraisal' summons images of school-type report forms, formal interviews and a slight unease for the appraisee who may perceive the exercise as threatening. Yet, to be effective the process can also be simple. It is perfectly possible to operate a performance review without forms, using a simple letter summarising the outcomes and agreements during the interview. The key to success is to match the system to the needs of those being appraised. Many practices have stable teams of staff with several years service and experience – they are not going to be motivated by a form that tells them they are judged as 'B minus' in telephone answering. A more appropriate route would be a letter to all staff explaining when the appraisals will be taking place, an outline of the interview topics and an invitation for each person to consider their own strengths, weaknesses, aspirations and training needs. The interview needs to be in a calm, undisturbed environment and followed by a written summary, one copy for the personnel file and one for the individual. In this way the practice manager can develop an atmosphere of working 'with' the team, not restricting performance discussions to when things go wrong! General practice has an advantage over a larger business in this respect because the manager can design a tailor-made system geared totally towards motivation.

Done well, the annual performance review can identify unrealised potential and skills that the practice can harness.

Discipline

No one enjoys disciplining a colleague; it highlights a failure of one or more of the following: comprehension, ability, communication, leadership or commitment. Curiously, the major issues are easier to deal with than the minor ones. Should a member of staff breach a patient's confidentiality, the manager's and partners' reactions will be swift and potentially result in a dismissal. In view of the gravity of the situation they will also take legal advice to ensure that they handle the dismissal fairly. Fortunately, this type of situation happens rarely; it is the more routine circumstances that cause a disproportionate amount of disruption. Take, for example, the receptionist who is constantly late by just a few minutes. The temptation is to leave well alone, working on the principle that a few minutes hardly matters. The longer term effects are more considerable. First, the other receptionists may decide that what is good for one is good for all and may also start arriving late. Secondly, the practice manager may be accused of favouritism because one person is allowed to deviate regularly from their working hours without comment. Thirdly, the group discipline declines and other small transgressions may develop. For all of these reasons the routine maintenance of standards must be upheld. The manager's role here is clear; they must identify the required standards and their own credibility and professional respect demands that they uphold them firmly, but sensitively.

Evidence-based management

The inclusion of a non-clinician in the practice decision-making core group has had enormous benefits. Instead of decisions based on gut reaction, we see decisions increasingly based on evidence. We have all heard sweeping statements about workload that are unchallenged, largely because no one really knows the true picture. For example, the partner who refuses to take any additional responsibilities because they have the highest number of elderly and consequently the greatest number of home visits. Managers can be quite unpopular when they audit workload and shoot the odd sacred cow! Most conflicts within partnerships revolve around workload, finance and the direction of the practice. Therefore, if the practice manager can undertake detailed analyses the foundation for making a major decision is much firmer and the correct choice is more likely to be made. This research may not be exclusively in-house; for example, reviewing a salary policy may include approaching other local practices or employers to establish a competitive rate of pay. In evidence-based medicine there are a large number of documents available for specific issues (e.g. drug therapies); this may not be quite so true of management, but there are many organisational models outside the NHS that can be applied to general practice.

Isolation

Earlier, the flexible and independent status of a practice manager was seen as a strength, but for the individual there is a disadvantage – feeling isolated. No one else in the practice has quite the same situation when it comes to discussing a problem. The manager cannot go to the staff as that would be disloyal and expose potential personal weaknesses. To go to the partners and express uncertainty about handling something takes courage, especially as the partners are also the employers. There is no one else in the practice doing the same job or at the level within the hierarchy. So where does a troubled manager go to seek guidance and discuss an idea? Not surprisingly, managers have found their own solution in the formation of managers' groups. Some are nationally recognised organisations which offer advice, newsletters and training courses to their members. Others opt for a more informal approach, meeting regularly at lunchtimes to discuss current issues and offering mutual personal support.

> In 1985 there were five practice managers in South Buckinghamshire who got together on an informal basis once a month, by 1995 the group had grown to twenty-seven.

These groups, formal or informal, are invaluable to practice managers. It allows a forum to seek and pool information, exchange examples of good practice, attend educational sessions and find an empathic ear for personal difficulties in a totally confidential environment. One group set up a system to inform each other when a staff member resigned and they were not suitable for re-employment elsewhere. In an area where there are several practices in close proximity this was a definite advantage, especially as managers tend to look kindly on people with previous experience of the NHS. Other groups combine their resources and run training courses for reception and administration staff very effectively.

Continuing personal development

The national groups, the Institute of Health Services Management (IHSM), the Association of Managers in General Practice (AMGP) and the Association of Medical Secretaries, Practice Administrators and Receptionists (AMSPAR), have all developed training courses that result in a certificate or diploma in management. They also stage annual conferences, open to members and non-members, where managers from all parts of the country can meet, hear presentations from leading health professionals and participate in workshop discussions. For those people who find educational time away from the practice difficult there are distance-learning packages available, where the projects are work related and can be combined with a busy working life. All of these things assist a manager in keeping up to date and, in turn, relaying information and suggestions back to the practice. The opportunities for continuing professional development are not restricted to the organisations mentioned above as many health authorities are delivering management courses in response to the comments and requests of practice managers in their geographical area.

As yet, there is no common entry standard for practice managers. Vacancy advertisements may state 'previous experience preferred' or 'a certificate or diploma from AMGP or AMSPAR would be an advantage', but there is not a defined package of skills and competencies that applies to all posts. The health authorities partly address this issue by asking practices to submit a 'person specification' with the application for salary funding. This secures local, but not national, standards for newly appointed managers. The titles given also vary (e.g. 'business manager', 'executive manager' and 'general manager'), all designed to give a more accurate indication of the level of responsibility. The core tasks remain the same, but the emphasis may be different.

Currently, a manager is responsible for their own professional development. The onus is on the individual to find an appropriate course or seminar and then seek the partners' approval for funding and time away from the practice. If the practice manager is regularly appraised and certain training needs have been identified, the process is a straightforward one. However, when personal objectives have never been agreed the manager is in danger of attending the wrong type of training, or becoming complacent about his or her own training needs. Funding is always a stumbling block, but every practice has a training budget to partly offset the costs.

> Sadly, there are still instances of managers taking their holiday entitlement to attend courses and funding them personally.

Another educational avenue for managers is the range of books available on all aspects of their role. Some, like *The handbook of practice management*, offer guidance on what to do and how to do it. The regular updates ensure that the reader is aware of new NHS policies and their implications. In addition, there are titles dealing with specific aspects (e.g. finance and computing). The practice library should reflect the needs of the entire team and include management books that are not directly related to general practice, but more generic management techniques (e.g. team building and personnel).

The economic climate of recent years and the restructuring of many major companies have resulted in a higher calibre of applicant than could have been anticipated 15 years ago. In the job market there are senior managers from financial institutions, multinational companies and ex-service personnel. The salaries offered to general practice managers have also become more attractive and an annual income of between £22k and £28k has become the norm, while for very large practices a salary of over £30k is not unusual. The media spotlight on NHS management has raised the awareness that it is a career option. The general fear is that such a 'high-flier' will not be content with practice management for more than a few years, rather than perceiving the appointment as an opportunity to bring in new thoughts and approaches.

> Recently, a practice in Norfolk advertising for a practice manager at a salary of £25k received 120 applications. They included a high percentage of candidates with professional qualifications, such as banking and financial management, many had taken advanced computer courses, one had an MBA and one was a solicitor.

As the overall performance of practice management increases there is a desire to harness these skills in other areas of primary care and find ways to communicate examples of good practice to lower achieving practices.

Extending practice management beyond the practice

Practice managers on assessment visits

In the Oxford Region, the assessment of new trainers and the re-approval of existing trainers and their practices for general practice vocational training had evolved into a peer group review. Since 1984, every trainer has been invited to participate in assessment visits. The visiting team of three was led by a team leader, usually a course organiser or an associate adviser. The visit itself was detailed, took a whole day, and resulted in a comprehensive report covering all aspects of the practice and the standard of teaching delivered by the trainer. Part of the assessment included a review of the organisational systems, administration and management, based on the concept that a training practice should offer an appropriate model in these areas as well as the clinical ones. In 1992, it was suggested that by adding an experienced manager to the assessing team several things might be achieved. The first was to free time for the trainers to undertake a more detailed review of the trainer's educational abilities, including feedback on video-recorded consultations and tutorials. The second was to improve the quality of information gained about the organisation and decision-making process in the practice. The third was to offer an opportunity for peer review and informed feedback to the non-clinical members of the primary healthcare team. In order to test the feasibility of including practice managers in the assessment process, it was essential to run a pilot study. To this end, five experienced practice managers, who were deemed to have good interpersonal skills, joined an assessing team and participated in visits. On the first few visits the practice managers simply observed and began to formulate ideas on how their skills could be best used. As their confidence and familiarity with the assessment criteria increased, they gradually assumed responsibility for observing and commenting upon the reception procedures and talking with the practice manager about general organisation. After 12 months the 'pilot' managers gave a presentation to the annual team leaders' study day, fielded their questions and listened to their feedback. The team leaders unanimously accepted the concept of adding practice managers to the assessing team.

Once the principle had been agreed the practicalities needed to be determined, together with some criteria that would secure a uniform approach. The criteria were simple: to be eligible a practice manager had to have two years experience in their post and be given a written reference by their training partner and a course organiser or existing manager already on the scheme. Once a practice manager was nominated they accompanied an experienced manager on two training visits. The first was to act purely as an observer and at the end they were debriefed by the experienced manager. On the second visit the nominated manager took the lead, was observed and again they were debriefed by the experienced manager at the end of the visit. Pending positive responses from both team leaders and accompanying practice managers, the new manager was accepted onto the scheme.

The original managers met regularly and designed a checklist of points to include under each heading of the visiting assessors' report, excluding clinical and the trainer's personal teaching ability. This ensured that the team leaders could delegate tasks appropriately throughout the course of the assessment visit and be confident about the range and quality of information that the practice manager would gather. The only reservation shared by visiting practice managers was that they would be asked to make judgements on clinical records. Here, the group felt that their role, if any, was one of statistical collection, not comment about quality or completeness.

The whole exercise has been evaluated and the overwhelming response of all parties, including the visited team, has highlighted the benefits.

As far as practice management was concerned this scheme offered an excellent development path for the managers who were eligible to participate. To spend a day in another practice and discuss their decision-making forum, organisational methods, examine channels of communication and the educational opportunities offered by the primary healthcare team to the GP registrar is a privilege. The whole team of visiting managers, without exception, had to handle each visit with sensitivity and maturity. The professional credibility of the scheme could have been destroyed by one manager behaving inappropriately. It also allowed for a general raising of management standards as good ideas and new insights were shared and the visiting managers were available to offer advice to newly appointed ones.

The Oxford Region's New Trainers' Course

To be approved as a trainer in the Oxford Region a GP must attend modules 1, 2 and 3 of the New Trainers' Course. Module 1 concentrates on preparing a practice for training, and explores the management of change to meet the training criteria, setting objectives and making plans. These are all management issues and since 1993 the course has been run with management tutors alongside clinical tutors. Practice managers have also been invited to attend with their prospective training partners, partly as an educational exercise for them but also to give the new trainer support in trying to attain the required standards of organisation.

Vocational training schemes

The appreciation of the need for management skills for future general practitioners has developed considerably, indeed, the Member of the Royal College of General Practitioners (MRCGP) examination now includes questions on management issues. The transition from registrar to partner can be traumatic and the anxieties rarely relate to treating patients, but to becoming accepted by the partnership team and additional financial and management responsibilities. Many course organisers use experienced practice managers to lead a teaching session at the local day release scheme to address this area of GP registrar learning.

What are the expectations of today's practice managers?

We cannot recruit and retain high calibre managers within general practice unless they are given a challenging role. The responsibilities and degree of autonomy must be in keeping with the salary and title. For this reason, employing a professional manager can be quite threatening. Some partnerships know that they need to be 'managed', but the reality of handing over a large chunk of their traditional authority can be difficult. Usually, this is a very short-term problem and a capable manager will quickly prove that such trust and confidence is not misplaced. Yet, practice management still does not have a defined career path; indeed, they are already the most senior member of the non-clinical team. There is no promotion to strive for, no perks such as a company car, and they will be well aware of the financial restrictions of staff salary budgets so large increases are out of the question – but are they?

Practice managers as partners?

The *Red Book* does not allow for anyone other than an approved GP principal to be recognised as a partner. Yet we are seeing an increasing number of managers offered partnerships. Until the recent taxation changes the phrase 'jointly and severally liable' discouraged managers from accepting a partnership, even if it was offered. That inhibiting factor has now been removed. It is still possible to offer partnership status in the form of profit sharing or a financial interest in the practice. These steps are not to be taken lightly and legal advice to produce a suitable agreement must be obtained. To the manager it probably formalises their real position, in other words, their commitment to maintain a profitable unit and involvement in every major decision.

When fundholding ends?

The change of government and the recent White Paper *The new NHS* have introduced an element of uncertainty about the future direction of general practice. The fund managers have been financed by the management allowance and when individual practice funds cease, so will the allowance. Many practices have benefited from the influence of new management skills sponsored by fundholding, yet they may be unable to afford to employ them. The fund managers have also gained an understanding of the NHS, and general practice in particular, which makes them a desirable commodity. The potential impact of this is twofold: there will be a pool of experienced managers seeking alternative employment in the more general field of practice management or within business management in secondary care and general practitioners may have to face dealing with mass redundancies of fundholding staff.

The impact of primary care groups on practice managers

The creation of primary care groups (PCGs) can be interpreted by some fundholding practices as a natural progression of the original scheme. The ability to take advantage of economies of scale by pooling resources and skills, yet reflecting accurately the needs of the local patient profile makes sense. For others, this is extremely threatening and unworkable. There are some practices who have difficulty in gaining consensus agreement over major issues among themselves, let alone gaining agreement with other practices. No matter what the personal views may be, to belong to a PCG is not an option, it is compulsory. Therefore, we must deal with the reality of the situation and the managers are thrust into the position of 'change agents' and implementers. At the time of writing there are definitely more questions than answers and further guidance is awaited on resourcing and information technology. However, there are a number of priorities already emerging that require the attention of practice management:

- What roles will individual members of the practice play within the PCG?
- What impact will these responsibilities have on the practice timetable and workload?
- Reading all the relevant documentation to assimilate the information and present it to the partnership for discussion
- To keep the staff informed and deal with individual concerns sensitively
- To plan for redundancies, if these are likely, and liaise with the appropriate bodies to ensure that these are dealt with legally and fairly
- What administration will be required at practice level to support the PCG?
- Is there spare accommodation that could be rented to the PCG?
- How will the practice elicit the views of patients?

Some practice managers will welcome this challenge and see it as an opportunity to develop their skills within a larger group. It is a learning experience where certain management techniques, like leadership, will be critical to the success of any PCG.

The future structure of the primary healthcare team

We can no longer assume that the traditional structure of general practice will continue. There are debates about the self-employed status of GPs and the possibility of a salaried service. The NHS contract with health authorities and patients may change, with the doctors acting as providers for primary care. We have definitions of 'core' and 'non-core' services which will inevitably shift some secondary care services into primary care (suitably funded, of course!). There are nurse practitioners who will enjoy a similar clinical status to GPs, and many practice teams have been extended to include other health professionals, such as physiotherapists and counsellors. Practices are working together more readily, enhanced by the development of co-operatives for out of hours cover and purchasing initiatives.

> In 1985, if a partner retired or resigned, they would have automatically been replaced by another partner working the same pattern and number of hours. By 1995, it could no longer be assumed that a direct replacement was the only option. Discussions centred around workload and cost, with the result that some full-time partners were replaced by a half-time partner and a full-time practice nurse or additional administrative staff.

There are external changes that will have a bearing on the way primary care is delivered, and a current political, economic, social, technological, legal and ecological (PESTLE) analysis of general practice is shown in Box 4.2.

At first sight, some of the issues seem irrelevant to general practice, but consider the increasing number of people working from home, linked to their offices by computer modem links and fax machines. If the trend continues we may be faced with reviewing our surgery hours; perhaps evening and early morning consultations will become obsolete if more patients can attend during the

Box 4.2: The PESTLE analysis

Political
- Change in government policies
- Future of fundholding and the purchaser/provider split
- Taxation rates and employers' National Insurance contributions
- Investment in education and training.

Economic
- Accountability for NHS costs
- Level of NHS resources and funding
- Confidence in the economy
- Investment in new premises
- Deregulation.

Social
- Demographic changes
  - increase in the number of elderly
  - birth rate
- Increased patient expectation
- Rise in cynicism
- Rise in consumerism
- Increasing litigation.

Technology
- The internal effects of computerisation
  - the paperless practice
  - audit potential
- Increase in homeworking
- The information super-highway!
- Evidence-based medicine.

Legal
- Health and safety
- Employment
- Accounting procedures
- Product liability
- Industrial relations.

Ecological
- Recycling
- The 'green' revolution
  - demand for natural medicines
  - homeopathy
- Animal testing.

day. Similarly, the Internet allows access to research papers about specific medical conditions and effective medication to patients as well as doctors. It is not impossible for a patient to be better informed than their GP!

Summary

The only thing we can be sure of in general practice is constant change. Some are external, like those in the PESTLE analysis, and some are internal to the medical profession created by a constant striving to deliver the best possible care to patients. Each year we see advances in diagnostic equipment and less invasive surgical procedures.

At the birth of the NHS in 1948 I feel sure that no one anticipated that transplant surgery and joint replacements would become routine operations, free of charge to the recipients.

These changes need not be negative and threatening, they all offer general practice a chance to review their policies and working methods. The criticisms of unwelcome centrally imposed changes have largely been about the way new health policies have been introduced, not about the motives or desired outcomes. Many of the changes have been positive, and no one would deny that setting targets in 1990 for cervical cytology and childhood immunisations improved the overall uptake for these services.

The practice manager is ideally placed to act as the change agent by exploring the options and opportunities and translating theories into action plans. Resources will never be unlimited and we must gain the maximum potential from all of them, especially the primary healthcare teams. To maintain the most enviable health service in the world we must foster a feeling of pride in what general practice can achieve, which will in turn prompt innovations and a constant quest for excellence. This must come from the grass roots of the medical profession and it will need to be managed effectively. The future of management in general practice has never been more challenging, or rewarding.

Further reading

1 Belbin M (1981) *Management teams – why they succeed or fail.* Butterworth Heinemann, Oxford.

2 Hasler J, Bryceland C, Hobden-Clarke L and Rose P (1991) *The handbook of practice management.* Longman, London.

3 Johnson N, Hasler J, Hobden-Clarke L and Bryceland C (1997) The role of a practice manager in training assessment visits. *Education for General Practice,* **8**: 128–34.

4 Maslow A H (1970) *Motivation and personality* (3e). Harper and Row, New York.

5 Pringle M, Bilkhu J, Dornan M and Head S (1991) *Managing change in primary care.* Radcliffe Medical Press, Oxford.

6 Weightman J (1996) *Managing people in the Health Service.* Institute of Personnel and Development, London.

5

Making change happen: developing primary healthcare teams

Peter Havelock and Theo Schofield

Outline

- The development of primary healthcare
- The elements of effective teamwork
- The defining of primary healthcare teams
- The principles of change management
- External influences on primary healthcare
- Examples of producing change

Introduction

The evolution from general practice largely caring for individuals when they are ill to primary care teams providing healthcare for their whole population has been the most dramatic change in the National Health Service in the past 25 years. It has not always been comfortable for those involved, particularly at times when they have not felt in control of events, but it has also been exciting and rewarding to have been part of this remarkable development. This chapter will describe some of our experience as doctors working in our own practices, and some of our involvement in projects aiming to promote change in wider practice.

The developing concept of primary healthcare

The National Health Service has always had two guiding aims: to enable everyone to have access to the medical care they need irrespective of their income; and to improve the health of the population. It is clear that the first involves transferring the question of affordability from the individual to the state, and a system of healthcare that involves universal access to low cost, low technology care, and restricted access to specialist care is essential to achieving this aim. General practitioners in this country have also valued the referral system as a guarantee of their professional role as family doctors to everyone, not just those that cannot afford specialists, as is the case in many other countries.

The opportunities in this structure for the GP are considerable. Not only can the practice provide personal and continued care for a list of registered patients with the personal rewards that this can bring, but there is also the expectation and the need for as many new services as possible to be provided in this accessible but low cost environment. But here is the first challenge. Developing an effective primary care team and the services they provide requires working with larger numbers of people, learning new skills, adopting new technologies, developing new relationships and, above all, changes in our roles.

Chronic disease management in general practice, the care of frail elderly people in their own homes, community care of the mentally ill, open access to investigations, earlier discharge and day care in hospitals are all part of this growth of the services provided, which in turn has led to expanded community nursing teams, the growth of the practice nurse, computerisation of records and many other changes that are now easily taken for granted.

Achieving the second aim of promoting health is even more difficult. There is a clear relationship between social inequality and health and part of the thinking behind the NHS was that equal access to health services would help to correct this. Again it is now easy to take for granted the importance of ensuring that everyone receives childhood immunisations, family planning, antenatal care, support for child rearing and appropriate screening for treatable conditions. However, the job description of a GP in *The future general practitioner* in 1972 did not include responsibility for the care of the registered population, but now this is a central part of the work of a primary healthcare team.[1]

Social inequalities in health, however, persist, and there is continued debate about the reasons for this. In part it may be due to what Julian Tudor Hart described as the 'inverse care law', that health services are provided in inverse proportion to their need, and it remains a challenge to ensure equity in the standards of primary care services, and that they do meet the needs of their population.[2]

In the past ten years much attention has been given to the effects that smoking habits, diet, alcohol and physical activity have on health, and doctors and primary care teams have been urged to attempt to advise their patients to adopt healthier lifestyles. All the evidence now is that this has a limited effect and that more attention should be given to the causes of ill health in the population.[3]

It is easy to conclude that this is beyond the GP's remit, but a broader concept of primary healthcare builds on its strength of being located in the community to identify the health needs of their population and to work with other individuals and agencies to help to meet them. This model has been described by Nigel Stott,[4] from an international perspective, and by Julian Tudor Hart[5] from his experience in the community of Glycorrwyg. It does involve a 'new kind of doctor', and in particular a new kind of relationship with one's community. The essential ingredient is to build on the strengths of individuals and communities and to enable them to take more control over the factors that affect their health. If communities are taking more control, then doctors and other professionals working in primary care need to accept that they will have less, which may be uncomfortable.

The rest of this chapter will concentrate on two areas of development: the creation of effective primary care teams providing a wide range of services, and the orientation of primary care to establish the needs of their population, and to work with other agencies in the community to meet them.

Elements of effective teamworking

Teams and teamworking have been an accepted part of industry and commerce for many years: sales teams, project teams, design teams, production teams, etc. A great deal has been written about the elements of effective teams. There is general agreement about the factors needed to produce an effective team.[6] These need to be considered, developed and personalised by the group of people as they come together to form their team

A sense of shared purpose: the vision

In general practice this may be considered as obvious – the best possible care for the patient. Few members of primary healthcare teams (PHCTs) would disagree with this as a vision for primary healthcare, but how it is brought about and what is meant by best possible care can have very different meanings to different people. The following are contrasting views about general practice that can lead to very different visions of primary healthcare:

- Care based on research evidence compared with care based on experience alone
- The GP as the undisputed leader of the team compared with recognising leadership in team members
- Education based on reading and workshops compared with learning by doing.

So often, PHCTs have not spent the time, effort or emotional energy discussing and developing a shared vision and achieving the shared sense of purpose needed for effective teamworking.

A definable membership

Primary healthcare teams vary in the types of people who are seen to be included in the team. It is important that all members of the team are clear about the roles of the other members. The roles played by individuals in the team are made up of the professional skills and personal attributes brought in by the individual. For example, the health visitor brings to the team the skills of child care, health promotion and care of the elderly. An individual health visitor may bring group skills while another might contribute the skills of individual counselling. Time spent discovering each other's skills and knowledge and defining roles based on those attributes is time well spent.

Group consciousness

To function effectively a team needs to define working patterns and an individual's responsibilities within the team. An example that most people can relate to is timekeeping. Most doctors have all felt the frustration when the team has agreed to meet at 1 p.m. and one or two of the key members have still not arrived after half an hour. Most of the rules are unwritten and often unspoken which means that the members can be unclear about them. It helps considerably if the rules and responsibilities are overt and clear so that everybody knows and understands them.

Interdependence

A team is more than a group of independent people pursuing their own agendas. Time needs to be set aside for the members of the practice to relate to each other. In a busy general practice it is easy to act independently, have expectations of other members of the team, but not give them time to find out about those expectations. It is easy to say to a computer operator 'Please get out the data for the practice report', but unless time is spent defining what is needed, discussing the best means of presentation and ensuring understanding, the job is very unlikely to be completed satisfactorily. Although a team is made up of individuals some autonomy needs to be sacrificed for the greater benefit of the whole team. The time spent and the individual autonomy lost are more than made up for by the time saved and the sense of group membership of a high performing team that is fostered.

Leadership

The primary healthcare team needs leadership. This is not control, not ordering about, not a boss, but a leader. John Adair in *Not bosses but leaders*[7] defines the leader as having the ability to influence others to achieve a common goal. Some of the qualities of a good leader are:

- integrity: the quality that makes people trust you – personal wholeness
- enthusiasm
- warmth
- calmness
- being tough but fair.

Further help in defining the characteristics of leadership are offered in the excellent book by Rosemary Stewart *Leading in the NHS*.[8] She lists the characteristics as:

- pointing the way forward: having a vision of what is to be achieved within the practice
- symbolising what matters: a leader shows clearly by his action what he cares about
- getting others to share your ideals
- creating a pride in the organisation: getting people to identify with their part of the practice and feel proud of where they work. Pride is linked to achievement and high standards
- making people feel important: people have more energy and will set themselves higher standards if they think that they, and what they do, matter
- realising people's potential: effective leaders provide an environment within which people's energies are released and they feel able to innovate

- self-sufficiency: being a leader can be lonely so the leader must learn to accept himself and rely on himself.

The leadership of the practice needs these qualities. They are not necessarily the qualities that come with a medical training or a management course. It does not automatically follow that the doctor in the PHCT provides the leadership, although leadership is more likely to come from the partners because of their financial and time commitment to the practice.

If there is no leadership, effective teamwork is most unlikely to be achieved. If the partners in the practice do not have the wish or the qualities to provide leadership they must encourage the practice manager or another to provide the leadership and guidance to the PHCT.

Communication

Communication between the members of the team is the cement between the building blocks. Without effective communication between the individual members of the teams the other aspects of teamwork fall apart. This communication needs to be effective whatever the medium and whatever the situation: practice meetings, informal discussions, written communication within or outside the practice.

What is a primary healthcare team?

The constituent members of the PHCT can vary as much as the number of times the question is asked: 'Who should be in the team?'. Some teams include the community pharmacist, chiropodist, practice gardener, and cleaner, while others are limited to the doctor, nurse and receptionist. Each practice defines for itself the membership of its PHCT depending on the resources and situation locally and the attitude and values of the constituent members.

In an editorial in the *British Medical Journal*, Pearson and Jones questioned the value of the large PHCT and suggested that effort should be made to look at smaller teams in the practice. They concluded: 'Encouragement to develop a rather nebulous primary healthcare team should be replaced by an emphasis on cohesive multidisciplinary working to achieve clearly established aims and objectives.'[9]

To try and encourage teamwork in a group of more than ten is very difficult. In most practical circumstances the practices divide up into functional groups:

- **The whole primary care team** This group share a common aim and a common group of patients. Meeting together provides the forum for smaller teams which have been working on different aspects of the practice. Getting together may be rare, such as at a review meeting around the practice report, or at the annual social function.
- **The management team** This usually includes the doctors and practice manager but sometimes also fund manager, senior practice nurse or senior receptionist. The vision and leadership for the practice comes from this group although the composition may vary from practice to practice.
- **The administrative team** This comprises those people in the practice without direct clinical care: the receptionist, secretary, accounts clerk and other administrative employees. Many of these jobs are dependent on each other and require close co-operation within the group.
- **The practice nurse team** There has been a large increase of employment of practice nurses in general practice with a need for co-operation and joint working. They need to be aware of 'who does what' and have common policies between themselves.
- **The attached staff team** Health visitors and district nurses bring different skills but often the biggest barrier to working as a single nursing team is their separate employment. Changes in the organisation of primary care will, it is hoped, diminish the distinction between the practice nurse team and the attached staff team.
- **Subject project teams** In practical working terms, it is in much smaller groups that the PHCT works effectively. These are groups set up to achieve a task or project, for example, clinical matters

such as an *asthma team*: the doctor, practice nurse and a record clerk; or the *antenatal team*: midwife, health visitor and doctor; or around administrative subjects (e.g. the *practice report*; practice manager, doctor and audit assistant); or the *patient participation group*: patient representatives, manager, senior receptionist, doctor. These teams can be set up for a limited time to achieve a certain task or can be ongoing.

- **Patient care teams** These are small groups focused together on the care of a specific patient. They are continually developed and disbanded depending on the health of the patient. Examples might be a patient dying at home when the team might be the district nurse, doctor, Macmillan nurse and the local group of volunteers, or a patient with postnatal depression when the team might be the health visitor, community psychiatric nurse and the doctor.

Whatever the constituent members of these teams and whatever their function, the elements of effective teamworking need to be considered.

Recently, West and Poulton questioned the effectiveness of these teams in practice by comparing them with other teams in and outside the health service. They said: 'Our quantitative and qualitative research suggests that a major problem in primary healthcare teamwork is the difficulty of developing clear shared objectives amongst the different professionals involved'.[10]

Needs-led primary care

The idea that primary care services should meet patients' needs sounds self-evident, but in fact contains a number of difficult components. The first is that the way the practice works should be planned to suit the patients and not the interests of those providing the service. Why do most appointment systems ensure that there are always patients waiting for doctors rather than a doctor always available for patients? Also consider whether some of the things the practice does are because they are new and interesting, rather than the best way to use time and resources for the benefit of the patients.

If the standard definition of a need as the ability to benefit from health services is acceptable, then this raises the issue of whether many of the interventions really do benefit the patients. The difficulty, particularly in primary care, is that the evidence for much of that work may not be available and that the process of obtaining and appraising evidence over the whole range of topics is time consuming and daunting.

Patients may have health problems, but do not need health services to solve them. An older woman who cannot do her own shopping because of pain in her hip does not immediately equate this with a need for a hip replacement. She may be helped more by ground-floor housing, buses that are easier to get on and off, or a local good neighbours' scheme. If she takes her problem to the doctor, or if it is detected by the team's surveillance programme, how can the team react? It could be medicalised, with a prescription or referral on to a waiting list, or the team could put her in contact with local services, advocate on her behalf, or even work with others in the community to develop the good neighbours' scheme if it is apparent that there is a need for one.

The team could also reflect that her problem may have been caused by her being overweight and having limited access to physical activity in earlier life and work with their community to promote physical activity. One of the reservations professionals have about seeking out needs is the fear of raising expectations that cannot be met by limited resources, but primary care has the potential resources of the whole community if the practice chooses to identify and work with them.

How does the practice find out what the patients' health needs really are? One of the assumptions underlying the health service reforms and the idea of a primary care-led NHS is that GPs are well placed to do this, but it requires a systematic effort if this is not to become an exercise in replacing one professional group's opinion with another or, dare one suggest it, an attempt to divide and rule. The available methods have been reviewed in an Occasional Paper edited by Gillam and Murray,[11] and those that have a valuable use in practice include:

- *Anecdote* The comments of patients on their problems and the services they have received remain an important source of insight and can be the starting point for further exploration. It was the comments of young mothers and older people about the difficulty of getting in to the surgery that led to a rural transport scheme run by volunteers.

- *Use of census and other data* The census and the report of the Director of Public Health contain information on health priorities, the ethnic mix of the area, housing, employment and other factors affecting health that can be applied to the practice population.
- *Use of data routinely collected in the practice* There is a large amount of data held in the records and registers in the practice that can inform decisions about services. For example, the numbers of children, mothers and elderly people and health visiting, the numbers of patients with chronic diseases and practice nursing, and waiting lists and secondary care services.
- *Incidence rates* Many practices collect data on admissions, deaths and other events. Because these numbers can be converted to rates in the registered population comparisons can be made with other areas, even though the confidence that can be placed in small numbers may not be great. A high termination of pregnancy rate led to a reappraisal of family planning services and to work with the local school and youth clubs on teenage health.
- *Systematic surveys* The information collected in health checks and surveillance of patients aged over 75 can be aggregated to produce information about unmet needs (e.g. the number of people having difficulty with chiropody, hearing problems, bathing or doing their laundry). Again, part of the response to this is the provision of more health services, but this information can also be shared with social services and voluntary agencies for them to respond as well.
- *Focus groups* Discussions with small groups of patients sharing the same problems or experiences can be a very powerful and economical way of obtaining information about needs or services. One evening spent with a group of patients with diabetes led to considerable change in the way that their services were organised.
- *Rapid appraisal* This involves asking key informants in an area about their views on health needs and services. Many people

will have very different perspectives, from the organiser of the toddler group, the school, the police, the youth club, etc., and will also know about the strengths, capacities and sources of leadership in the community. This may be done in a limited way by existing members of the team, but a dedicated community development worker can make a real impact by establishing networks, identifying resources, and facilitating changes that can help a community tackle their own problems.

A final issue to be considered is the question of resources and priorities, and the role of primary care in deciding them. It has been argued that the doctor's role is to advocate on behalf of each individual patient, and that the GP should not be involved in making choices or the rationing of services in any way. On the other hand, it can be said that practices and teams have always been involved in rationing the numbers of staff and the way they use their time and their other resources, and that what is being asked now is that this should be done in a more explicit way and over a wider range of services. Unless the practice is well informed about the real needs of the patients it will not be able either to make the case for the resources that are required, or to plan and provide the primary care services that meet them.

Principles of change management

These are major changes in the way that general practice works and sees itself. How has this change been promoted and achieved? The structure of general practice, with individual or partnerships of doctors with 'independent contracts' with their health authorities, and members of the potential primary healthcare team being employed by different agencies, makes the management of change both from outside the practice and within it notoriously difficult. Horder *et al.* reviewed ways of influencing the behaviour of general practitioners and concluded that no single method was particularly effective.[12] However, there is an extensive literature on the management of change which has been used to develop the following set of approaches used and advocated in our own practices and in our work as leaders of a succession of projects in our health districts to promote team development.[13–15] Some of the principles that underlie these approaches are:

- Everyone in primary healthcare has great scope for 'opting out' in one way or another. The essential process is therefore based on persuasion and consent.
- There is often a tension between top-down agendas (e.g. *Health of the Nation* targets) and professionals' agendas for themselves and their patients. A process that recognises and seeks to meet both is more likely to be effective than a one-way process.
- In any change there will be many stakeholders. They need to be recognised and their views taken into account. Their permission may be all that is required but everyone needs to be valued.
- Consultation with those involved in any change improves the planning as well as helping to win co-operation.
- Individuals and practices vary in their need for help and the type of support they require to change. Provision therefore needs to be multifaceted, flexible and responsive to their needs.
- A combination of methods is more likely to be successful in bringing about change than any single intervention.
- Practices need to be offered a variety of tools that they can use for planning from which to choose.
- Some topics (e.g. communication skills, teamwork and attitudes) are often difficult to get discussed directly. It may be easier to link these with discussion of specific content.
- Delivery of patient care in general practice is virtually impossible without an effectively working PHCT and therefore team members and teamwork must be included in any intervention.

The irony is that these principles are very similar to those used by GPs when trying to help patients to change – establishing people's ideas and concerns, sharing information, agreeing plans and responsibilities and building relationships and responding to people as individuals – but they need to be learnt again when trying to produce change in practice.

The model of change that seems to describe best what happens in a district when a change is introduced is the 'diffusion of innovations' model of Everett Rogers.[16] Its strength is that it recognises that some practices will be early adopters and others later, but that this is a dynamic process that can be fostered and not a fixed division between those that will and those that will not change.

The external environment

It is possible to identify a number of particular events which have created the environment which has encouraged the development of primary healthcare to take place. It is likely that external events will continue to play a major part in shaping this environment:

- The 1966 Charter for General Practice which provided funding for practice staff and premises.
- Vocational training for general practice which provided broadly trained and well-motivated entrants to general practice.
- The attachment of community nurses to general practices to form PHCTs. This received powerful encouragement from the Cumberlege Report in 1986 which stated that: 'Nurses are at their most effective when working in well functioning primary care teams'. (Far less often quoted is the next sentence stating that: 'These are more often a concept than a reality'.)
- The series of Royal College of General Practitioners (RCGP) reports in 1980 on the scope of prevention and health promotion in primary care.
- The international health promotion movement which recognised the central role of primary care in tackling social inequalities in health, set targets for Health for All by the Year 2000, and which led to our own *Health of the Nation* targets.
- The 1990 Contract for general practice which included payments for health promotion. Its method of introduction, which flew in the face of virtually all the principles of effective change management, has meant that its only lasting effects are an improvement in child immunisation rates and a lingering resentment contributing to low morale and recruitment problems.

- Fundholding, which was introduced at the same time, was an opportunity to develop new services in primary care and to divert resources from secondary care. For a variety of reasons this has not happened as much as one might have expected.
- The change in the nature of health authorities so that they have a planning and service development responsibility for primary care, and an overview of the relationship between primary and secondary care.
- In 1997, the change of government produced the demise of fundholding and the rise of primary care groups, clinical governance and health improvement programmes.

The rate and number of these external changes are increasing so it therefore follows that primary healthcare needs to remain fit and able to respond in an appropriate and effective way.

Producing change in a district

The author's primary care team development work started in 1986 with the Wycombe Primary Care Prevention Project.[16] This was initially funded by the Regional Health Promotion Fund to develop health promotion, particularly the prevention of arterial disease. It was based on the facilitation model developed in Oxford, and throughout the project the work done by the facilitator in working with and meeting the needs of individual practice teams has been crucially important.[17]

The Project ran for ten years and during that time its agenda evolved considerably to meet national and local priorities (e.g. Health of the Nation), and to respond to the needs expressed by PHCTs themselves. The range of methods used to help individuals and teams has also expanded to include those described below.

Multidisciplinary study days

There have been a series of study days based at the three postgraduate centres within the county where practice teams come to work around a specific subject. Examples used are: *teenage health* – with a doctor, practice nurse and interested receptionist; *stop smoking*

– for practice nurse, health visitor and doctor; and a similar team for the *healthy eating* study day.

The days are designed around a mixture of theoretical inputs, communication skills development, strategic and tactical planning. It is hoped that the participants return to the practice with a clear idea of what they want to do, based on explicit evidence and the skills and methods of how they will implement them.

Residential team workshop: practice planning based on needs

This is an opportunity for small teams from practices, of four to six members, to come together for two days, identify an area of need within their population and plan care to meet that need. This is helped by inputs on: needs assessment; team dynamics; roles in teams; community development; planning; and effective meetings.

Many practices in the county have attended and the range of subjects that they have worked with has been wide: care of diabetic patients; ethnic minorities within the practice; non-smoking strategy; care of the elderly; patient access; reduction of mortality/ morbidity of ischaemic heart disease.

Practice away days

The health authority (HA) supports practices to take all the PHCT members out of the practice for a day to encourage strategic planning. The costs of the venue and facilitator are met by the HA and the primary care facilitator can assist with the administration and the identification of suitable people to help facilitate the day. The methods used vary considerably depending on the practice, but the emphasis is on developing a clear vision for the practice, identifying roles and responsibilities and encouraging effective communication.

Producing change in a county

Following the change in the remit of the Family Health Services Authority, and later the formation of a single Health Authority, there is now a clear commitment by the Buckinghamshire Health Authority to the development of primary care based on the PHCT. After wide consultation, a County Primary Care Strategy has been produced jointly by the health authority, local medical committee and the postgraduate department. This strategy gives priority to the development of high performing PHCTs and the document states under the heading 'Teams and organisations':

> Teams will exist for patient care that are functional task orientated, self-educating and who communicate effectively (with all parties) sharing information and looking after one another. Organisational structures will provide a framework for outlining roles and responsibilities providing vision, leadership and accountability.

There is recognition in the document that teams that both learn together and become involved in research develop a strength in their role as healthcare providers.

As part of the primary care strategy evidence-based dissemination is included. For each new development, a clear plan of how a new project should be disseminated and implemented is made based on the wealth of evidence in the literature concerning the adoption of innovations. This diffusion is managed by a multi-agency steering group, the Buckingham Primary Care Development Forum, made up from GPs, HA staff, nurses, patients groups, academic units, practice managers, and community trust staff. The forum is supported by the Executive and the Board of the Health Authority and its papers are widely circulated. The forum has the clear aims of networking throughout the county, dissemination of 'good practice' and identifying the needs for development and support of educators in the community.

There have been other activities within the county that have been part of the development of primary healthcare teams:

- *Development of nurse groups and practice manager groups* these empower the non-doctor members of the team and encourage the development of networks
- *Nurse prescribing pilot* encouraging the community nurse to take responsibility for a drug budget of limited prescribing
- *Practice nurse conference* a celebration of the wide range of activities of practice nurses and the development of new skills and aspirations.
- *Critical appraisal skills for practice workshop* to develop in all team members critical appraisal skills to encourage evidence-based practice.

- *Formation of the Buckinghamshire Primary Care Research Network* (Bucks ResNet) this is multidisciplinary in formation and membership, based in the Centre for Research in Primary Care at the local nurse training college. The activities include active teaching of research skills, workshops for early projects, supporting new projects, and Acorn Funding to encourage the writing of research proposals.
- *The use of the teaching network* the teaching networks within the county for both doctors and nurses are supported and encouraged to experiment with new ideas in their practices. They then become opinion leaders and role models for others who work locally within their neighbouring practices. Examples of this are commissioning groups, local continuing medical education groups, fundholding groups and out-of-hours co-operatives.
- *Celebration of success* there were three or four conferences in 1998 to celebrate the successes of various aspects of primary healthcare. There is encouragement to record each activity and there is a regular newsletter of development activities produced by the Bucks ResNet.

All these activities are followed up and co-ordinated by the primary care facilitators and the medical audit advisory group (MAAG) facilitators who work closely together using the skills of facilitation to identify the requirements for each practice to develop and to provide the expertise, skills or information that will help them move.

Regional support

Within the four counties of the Oxford Region there have been other activities that have encouraged the development of effective teams. These are described below.

Peer group visiting

There has been a close involvement, locally, with peer group visiting, dating back to the *What sort of doctor?* scheme in the early 1980s. This was developed locally into the peer group assessment of training practices.[18] This system has been very influential in developing effective teams within the training practices. There is a great emphasis within the visits of the late 1990s on the active involvement of the practice members in the teaching. This has the result that the team has to look at their development to meet this challenge. There is further encouragement within the area for GPs to become Fellows of the RCGP by assessment, an approach that encourages effective teamwork.

The learning practice: a multidisciplinary workshop
Another result of this emphasis on team rather than individual teaching was the cry from the non-training GPs and PHCT members that they needed help and support in developing their teaching skills. This has led to the very successful multidisciplinary workshop *The learning practice,* which encourages the development of teaching and learning within the practice. It also helps the GPs to achieve a developmental learning culture.

Close links with academic units and public health
These have been developed with the Department of Public Health and Primary Care in Oxford, and the link to the nurse academic network is through the Centre for Research in Primary Care at Brunel University and Luton University which provide basic and some post-basic training for the nurses. The regional co-operation between general practice and public health and the development of the Public Health Resource Unit have played a great part in the development of public health skills within general practice.

Conclusions

What are the principles behind these developments in general practice and what is applicable elsewhere?

The focus is on primary healthcare team development. Effective development needs structures and processes in place:

Structures

- Multidisciplinary planning

- Development of strong community networks in teaching and research
- Concentration on dissemination strategies for each activity
- Development of opinion leaders in the community throughout the area.

Processes

- Multiple activities that allow practices to use and choose different activities for themselves
- Generic skills development of community workers either medical or from within the population
- Involving as wide a group of people as possible.

Effective development needs

- Leadership and commitment
- Effective communication
- Involvement of all at an early stage, and taking the people with you
- Clear vision
- Regular review.

All those involved with primary care development, whether it is within the practice, in a district, region or country as a whole, need to keep in mind these essential elements of effective change.

Summary

- Primary care is changing and will continue to change rapidly and thus primary healthcare teams need to develop the skills to meet those changes
- There is a theoretical and evidence base for developing teams and bringing about effective change
- Although notoriously difficult to change, primary healthcare, managed correctly, can be encouraged to develop
- The principles of change management, although easy to define, are more difficult to put into practice.

References

1 Royal College of General Practitioners (1972) *The future general practitioner: learning and teaching.* British Medical Journal Publications/RCGP, London.

2 Hart J T (1971) The inverse care law. *Lancet,* **1**:405–12.

3 Ebrahim S and Davey Smith G (1997) Systematic review of randomised controlled trials of multiple risk factor interventions for the prevention of coronary heart disease. *British Medical Journal,* **314**:1666–74.

4 Stott N (1983) *Primary health care: bridging the gap between theory and practice.* Springer, Berlin.

5 Hart J T (1985) *A new kind of doctor: the general practitioner's part in the health of the community.* Merlin, London.

6 Havelock P B (1995) *Communication skills and teamworking in primary care.* Publishing Initiatives, Beckenham.

7 John A (1990) *Not bosses but leaders.* Kogan Page, London.

8 Stewart R (1989) *Leading in the NHS: a practical guide.* Macmillan, London.

9 Pearson P and James K (1994) The primary care non-team. *British Medical Journal,* **309**:1387–8.

10 West M and Poulton B (1997) A failure of function: teamwork in primary health care. *Journal of Interprofessional Care,* **11**:205–16.

11 Gillam S and Murray S (1996) *Needs assessment in general practice.* Royal College of General Practitioners, London.

12 Horder J, Bosanquet N and Stocking B (1986) Ways of influencing the behaviour of general practitioners. *Journal of the Royal College of General Practitioners,* **36**:517–21.

13 Deming W (1986) *Out of the crisis.* MIT Center for Advanced Engineering Study, Cambridge, MA.

14 Berwick D (1992) Continuous quality improvement in medicine: from theory to practice. *Quality in Health Care,* **1**:2–8.

15 Rogers E (1982) *Diffusion of innovations.* The Free Press, New York.

16 Havelock P, Schofield T and Tapsfield J (1994) Health promotion in primary care: the British perspective. *American Journal of Preventive Medicine,* **10**:33–5.

17 Fullard E, Fowler G and Gray M (1984) Facilitating prevention in primary care. *British Medical Journal,* **289**:1585–7.

18 Schofield T P C and Hasler J C (1984) Approval of trainers and training practices in the Oxford Region. *British Medical Journal,* **228**:538–40; 614–18; 688–9.

Further reading

Berwick D (1992) Continuous quality improvement in medicine: from theory to practice. *Quality in Health Care,* **1**:2–8.
This paper, when written, had a very different perspective on quality in health. The author introduced the ideas of total quality management in a clear way without the jargon so often associated with the subject. He concludes by challenging the doctors in the health service to follow the path of systematic improvement before they are taken over by the 'world of inspection'.

Hart J T (1985) *A new kind of doctor: the general practitioner's part in the health of the community.* Merlin, London.
A strongly recommended book for those either entering general practice or who are questioning their role as a general practitioner. Julian Tudor Hart challenges the status quo and suggests that general practitioners should define and meet the needs of their population.

Havelock P B (1995) *Communication skills and teamworking in primary care.* Publishing Initiatives, Beckenham.
A handbook for any primary team members who wish to develop their practice and team. It contains many useful and practical ideas together with references to the management literature for those who wish to take the subject further.

Rogers E (1982) *Diffusion of innovations.* The Free Press, New York.
An accumulated collection of the research evidence for the effective diffusion of an innovation. Reading the book emphasises that the problems of encouraging change in general practice are not new and the problems are so similar to managing change in so many environments.

Schofield T P C and Hasler J C (1984) Approval of trainers and training practices in the Oxford Region. *British Medical Journal,* **228**:538–40; 614–18; 688–9.
A paper which, though written in the 1980s, describes the effective introduction of the quality criteria for a group of general practitioner trainers, together with the method for effectively assessing those criteria. Both the criteria and the method of introduction are as valid today as they were when the paper was written.

Stewart R (1989) *Leading in the NHS: a practical guide.* Macmillan, London.
A fascinating book based on the author's experience and research with groups of potential leaders in the NHS. It contains many useful ideas and offers insights into leadership that are valuable for any primary healthcare team members who wish to influence change in their workplace.

6

Beyond audit: quality improvement methods for changing practices

Martin Lawrence

Outline

This chapter reviews developments in improving primary healthcare quality over the past 25 years. The point is particularly stressed that improving quality requires change, and so is an educational exercise. Developing audit separate from continuing education has impaired its effectiveness. Recent developments in quality improvement methodology, together with combined working between audit and continued education groups, as well as across disciplines, gives the prospect of renewed progress.

The chapters in this book are not intended to make direct reference to John Hasler, but in the field of quality assurance that is difficult if not impossible. By 1970, there was a great *quantity* of general practice being undertaken; the problem was to raise the *quality*. Raising that quality became the prime aim of everything that John did – and most of the developments in the Oxford Region were under his guidance or at his instigation. This chapter traces quality assurance over the past 25 years from a predominantly (though not exclusively) parochial viewpoint, and John Hasler's profound influence cannot be overlooked.

Beginnings: the New College course

In the early 1970s, primary care developments relied heavily on the Royal College of General Practitioners (RCGP). This was hardly surprising. University departments for postgraduate medical education were in their infancy, and much of their academic time was spent researching the general practice aspects of clinical medicine. The government and health authorities were not deeply concerned with general practice – the 1966 Charter was less than ten years old, family practitioner committees (FPCs) were largely bodies for payments and contracts, and a primary care-led National Health Service was over 20 years away.[1]

It has been one of the paradoxes of the RCGP that its very success has resulted in its *apparent* ineffectiveness. The College's development of vocational training has been taken over by the postgraduate medical education (PGME) structure; its pressure for improved academic research opportunity has resulted in active university departments; its drive for quality has led to the establishment of medical audit advisory groups (MAAGs) and health authority driven targets. The College's very success works itself out of a role.

In the 1970s, the RCGP was the main engine for quality improvement, and the Thames Valley faculty and North West faculty were vigorous and forward looking. Each had a visionary as chairman, John Hasler and Donald Irvine. Both were dedicated to the quality improvement of general practice.

In 1977, John Hasler proposed – and the author, as a principal of only three years' standing, was conscripted to run – a further education course for general practitioners, to be run by general practitioners. At the time this was a major departure. Following the 1966 Charter, GPs had been given allowances (section 63) to attend continuing education – but almost all was of the 'refresher course' variety, at which consultants gave talks on recent advances and GPs came and listened.

Standard setting

This course was to be different. Its name embodied its focus: *Towards better general practice.* Its prime aim was to be standard-setting, and the work would be done in small groups consisting of and led by GPs, although with some specialist resource support. Attenders were recruited three months in advance and mailed background reading matter and reading lists in order to enable them to prepare for the discussions. At the end of the three-day course each group would not only draw up a policy for care, but members would take resolutions as to what they would do on returning to practice in order to ensure change. The groups often agreed to meet, some months after the course, to review progress and evidence of change.

Performance review

It was also decided, long before the term 'audit' was in common use, that practices needed data on the basis of which to assess their performance and the impact of changes on outcome. A further advantage of the early recruitment of participants was that they were able to collect data which were then analysed prior to the course and used as a basis for discussion. At first this was done by the organisers, but the support of Douglas Fleming of the Birmingham Research Unit at the RCGP proved a major benefit in developing the methodology and demonstrating its effect. By 1983, the course had resulted in two published papers relating to audits carried out by participants and demonstrating improvement in practice outcomes.[2]

Results

The course, a residential two-to-three day event, was first held in 1978 and continued, using a fairly consistent format, until 1992. Although entitled *Towards better general practice,* it rapidly became known after its regular venue as *The New College course.*

The course affected a significant number of the Oxford Region's GPs. Over the first four years 196 doctors attended, 13% of the GPs in the Region – and they came from practices which included a third of all the Region's GPs. The GP working groups were able to draw up 'guidelines' for care applicable across practices. The guidelines were not perhaps as 'evidence based' as would be required in 1998 – but it was at least a start! We were able to show that in some areas at least it resulted in change. And participants developed a clear idea of some of the benefits – and problems – of audit. Not least, many participants found it a really enjoyable method of continuing medical education (CME) and of meeting colleagues. An Oxford University Press book, *Continuing care in general practice*, was published drawing heavily on the resources of the *New College course* working groups.[3]

The course methodology has a great deal in common with the methodology of 'quality circles', a widely favoured method of quality improvement and CME in several European countries. Experience from the course can still extensively inform the problems and potentials for quality circles, not least regarding the effect of combining data gathering and audit with methods to develop practice.

The 'quality initiative'

The 'quality initiative' of the RCGP was proposed and developed by Donald Irvine when Chairman of Council.[4] The proposal was that each GP should undertake two commitments:

1 To describe his or her current work and be able to say what services his or her practice provides for the patients

2 To define specific objectives for the care of patients, and monitor the extent to which these objectives are met.

It is interesting that the two aims of the quality initiative were just the same as the two main aims of the *New College course* (i.e. standard-setting and performance review). As an initiative one might say that it was not particularly successful since it was not widely adopted by college members, although most members of Council undertook the exercise. The requirements were perhaps too extensive and non-specific. On the other hand, it crystallised the requirements for audit of and accountability for the quality of care, and in a sense set the agenda for the succeeding ten years.

'What sort of doctor?'

What sort of doctor? (WHATSOD) was a complementary exercise to the quality initiative.[5] While the quality initiative exhorted GPs to undertake standard-setting and performance review, WHATSOD showed them how to do it. A first working party selected four areas of performance and practice and developed criteria for the essential attributes that a doctor needed in order to be an effective practitioner in each of the areas. A second working party (chaired by Theo Schofield, then John Hasler's Associate Regional Adviser in General Practice) developed a method of practice visiting to implement the performance review. The areas of performance were:

- Professional values – in relation to patients and the community; priorities for care; and the evolution of the practice
- Clinical competence
- Accessibility
- Ability to communicate – with patients, staff and colleagues.

Methods of assessment by practice visiting included:

- Study of a practice profile circulated in advance of the visit
- Observation of practice premises, facilities and functioning
- Discussion with the primary healthcare team members
- Inspection of clinical records
- Review of a video-recording of recent consultations
- Interviewing the doctor to elicit views and understanding – including discussion of data derived from patient records.

The doctors in practices who became involved in WHATSOD visits commented on how much they learned both from visiting and being assessed. The more comments were specifically related to the criteria, and the more they were based on specific information generated at the visit, the more valuable they were to the visiting doctors and the more likely they were to lead to change. Some practices reported quite major changes as a result of their visit.[1]

Avedis Donabedian attended some visits in 1984 and wrote of WHATSOD:[1]

> I'm impressed, challenged and deeply moved by it. This is a formulation unique, as far as I know, in the range, depth and richness of what it perceives quality of care to be; particularly so in its recognition that values are the source from which every other virtue must necessarily flow. It recognises the inter-relationship of the organisation of a practice and the practitioners' performance.
>
> 'What Sort of Doctor' is also admirable as a method of assessment. It demonstrates a commitment to measuring, even if imperfectly, that which is important rather than only that which can be precisely measured. It is also characterised by a delicate balance of directiveness and flexibility: while principles, objectives and criteria are unequivocally declared, the standards of performance that may be reasonably attained are subject to local adjustment through peers.

Despite this endorsement by such an authority, the WHATSOD method of evaluation has not been universally adopted. Partly, there is a reluctance of doctors to expose themselves to close scrutiny or to make judgements on their colleagues. Perhaps more significantly, it is not part of established CME, and is time consuming. Nevertheless, many of the principles and systems were clearly expressed, providing a firm base for further development of quality improvement in practice. In addition, the methods developed provided a starting point for the highly successful system of assessing Oxford Region training practices, as described below.

Practice team visiting

A development of WHATSOD has been to extend practice team visiting in 'What sort of practice?' This changed the focus from an individual doctor to the practice team, with visits arranged between pairs of practices. The core visiting team consists of a GP, practice nurse and practice manager, but can also include a district nurse, health visitor, and other clinical or clerical staff. An added benefit of this style of visiting is that it brings together the team, both as visitors and as those who have to present their work.

Vocational training in general practice: assessment of training practices

A major engine of change and improvement in general practice over the past 25 years has been the vocational training programme.[6] Started as an RCGP initiative in the 1960s it only became established and compulsory in 1981, at which time responsibility passed from the College to the departments of postgraduate medical education.

Vocational training has been a superb crucible within which to test quality improvement. Teachers receive a fee, and have the privilege of a trainee registrar working in their practices during the training year, so there is a major incentive to being approved for training. Moreover, there is protected time and finance for professional development – section 63 payments were retained for vocational training purposes even after the 1990 Contract.

This has been an opportunity seen clearly by John Hasler, who has been Regional Adviser in the Oxford Region since 1971. A sophisticated assessment system has been put in place, underpinned by clearly expressed principles to ensure that the assessment is effective in improving practice.

- The criteria against which trainers and their practices are assessed are clearly expressed. Indeed, they are written, available, and agreed by the trainers themselves
- All trainers are involved as assessors. This not only creates a feeling of ownership, but increases the learning opportunities of the assessment visit
- The assessment is to encourage development. Few practices 'fail' training visits, so the report is written to identify areas for development and improvement. Moreover, as practices improve, so the criteria and acceptable performance levels can be raised
- Resources are available to encourage practice and practitioner development. The postgraduate education department runs

regular courses for trainers, as well as courses specifically on communication skills and management.

The method and results of the programme have been reported, and are a model of quality improvement.[6] The system contains many of the principles of WHATSOD, and reflects the strengths reported by Donabedian. It particularly concentrates on what is important, not what is easily measurable. There are firm directive criteria – but there is also flexibility. Above all, there is a determination among trainers and training practices to improve, both to demonstrate excellence, and to retain their right to train.

Moreover, vocational training can develop as needs change – and assessment can drive the process. Although superb in educational method and in methods of process (communication skills, record-keeping, accessibility), many practices are presently felt weak in research skills and critical appraisal. This defect is being remedied as course organisers and trainers become involved in research method development and appraisal skills courses: the evolving assessment criteria will ensure that improvement passes on to registrars and so to future practitioners.

The audit experience

Each of the methods described above – the *New College course*, the quality initiative, WHATSOD, and vocational training assessments – was mediated through the CME system. Each of them used similar principles – to identify good practice, set standards and criteria, change practice, and measure activity to evaluate results. As we have seen, the effect on practice quality has been measurable and positive.

This process has been defined as audit and is frequently described as a cycle, as shown in Figure 6.1. Although initially voluntary and part of an educational initiative, in 1990 it was changed when the government decided to insist on audit as part of the 1990 GP Contract reforms. This was a brave plan to improve primary care quality by encouraging all practices and practitioners to begin to improve along the same lines as the motivated had been doing through the 1980s.

Plan care
implement change
Agree criteria
set target standards
Involve the
practice team
Choose topic
Evaluate information
performance *vs* targets
Observe practice
collect data

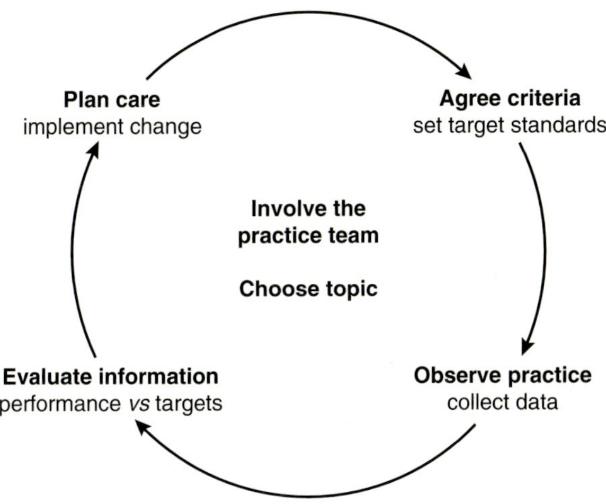

Figure 6.1: The audit cycle.

Unfortunately, two aspects of the audit initiative reduced its potential for success. First, it was introduced at the same time as a health-promotion policy, which imposed many clinical obligations on GPs, some of which were clearly futile and most of which were resented. Since these externally imposed criteria were associated with financial sanction, most GPs did comply, albeit with little enthusiasm. This left little time and energy for participation in self-motivated improvement and audit. Fortunately, most of these external constraints were removed in 1996, but not before general practice had suffered five years of severely low morale.

The other questionable aspect of the audit initiative was that MAAGs were set up to co-ordinate and oversee the exercise. MAAGs are semi-autonomous subcommittees of health authorities, and as such separate from the CME system. MAAGs have laid great emphasis on their confidentiality and independence from health authorities, but their financial dependence has led to increased joint working. This may be advantageous, since criteria for professional audit and health authority commissioning need to be kept in line. But it is also a disadvantage, since many GPs working on MAAGs are separate from those involved in the education system. Since change – the essence of quality improvement – is an educational exercise, this has undoubtedly resulted in a reduction of their effectiveness. A structure has been developed in which quality improvement and education are in separate compartments, to the detriment of both. (As an example, when in 1996 the RCGP launched guidelines for the management of back pain with a one-day conference, there was only one educationalist in the audience – and she left at lunchtime!)

Nevertheless, government sponsorship of audit through the early 1990s has led to clear benefits. The number of practices involved, undertaking audits which include setting standards and making changes, rose quickly. There are many examples of improvements in service delivery due to the implementation of audit, and in particular chronic disease management, especially of diabetes and heart disease, has been shown to be amenable to major improvement through audit.[7]

Satisfaction of MAAG criteria for audit can lead practices to feel that their quality improvement efforts are adequate. This is a problem since audit tends to be applied to a very narrow range of topics (mainly accessibility and chronic disease), and only a few members of each practice are usually involved. But of themselves these drawbacks hold some benefits, because they have driven practitioners to look for better methods of improving quality.

Guidelines

In the previous section it was stated that there were two major drawbacks to the audit initiative that impaired its success. There was perhaps a third – that the model did not adequately emphasise 'identify best practice' before the stage of setting standards. Indeed, the accepted model (*see* Figure 6.1) omits identification of best practice completely.

Many audits in the 1980s had been developed in which practitioners recorded items which were felt to be related to good practice; for example, frequency of hypnotic prescription, frequency of referral or number of home visits. Because there was no yardstick on which to base a standard, the feedback of data led to little change. General practitioners felt unhappy if their data showed them to be at the extreme end of a distribution, but comfortably content if somewhere near the middle.

Moreover, the plethora of external standards and targets demanded of GPs under the 1990 Contract led to a widespread demand from doctors to know the basis on which standards were set. It became apparent that before embarking on an audit it was essential to identify best practice – if there is no agreement on best practice then it is unhelpful to set up audits to see whether such practice is attained.[8]

Thus, the guideline movement was born of a need to set standards for practice. It was also born of an opportunity, the increased availability of data using electronic databases. Evidence-based medicine has become the vogue of the 1990s, and guidelines for practice based on firm evidence are important tools in quality improvement. Characteristics of guidelines that correlate with their likelihood of improving practice have been defined (*see* Box 6.1), together with the methods of implementation most likely to bring about change (*see* Box 6.2). Indeed, it has been clearly shown that it is not only the development and dissemination of guidelines that is important in producing change, but especially critical is the method of local implementation. A key early example was the North of England study, which showed that groups of GPs who developed guidelines for themselves changed, but that they did not change in response to guidelines developed by others.[9]

Quality improvement and total quality management

Thus, during the past 20 years, many strategies and techniques for quality improvement have been developed.[10] Most of them work, to an extent, but few work well on their own. Extensive studies at McMaster University[11] and a recent study in the UK[12] agree that education alone is the most effective change agent, but education alone only accounts for about a sixth of all changes. Most important is to have several influences working together.

Work derived from the total quality management (TQM) theory is suggestive of ways in which we in primary care can improve quality by using all the various techniques together. The principles are embodied in Figure 6.2, and have been more extensively summarised

Box 6.1: Desirable attributes of clinical guidelines

Attribute	*Explanation*
Validity	Guidelines are *valid* if, when followed, they lead to the health gains and costs predicted for them
Reproducibility	Guidelines are *reproducible* if, when given the same evidence and methods of development, another guideline group produces essentially the same recommendations
Reliability	Guidelines are *reliable* if, when given the same clinical circumstances, another health professional interprets and applies them in essentially the same way
Representative development	Guidelines should be developed by a process that entails participation by key affected groups
Clinical applicability	Guidelines should apply to patient populations defined in accordance with scientific evidence or best clinical judgement
Clinical flexibility	Guidelines should identify exceptions to their recommendations and indicate how patient preferences are to be incorporated in decision-making
Clarity	Guidelines must use unambiguous language, precise definitions and user-friendly formats
Meticulous documentation	Guidelines must record participants involved, assumptions made, and evidence and methods used
Scheduled review	Guidelines must state when and how they are to be reviewed (under two separate circumstances – the identification or not of new scientific evidence or professional consensus)

Adapted from *Guidelines for clinical practice: from development to use.* ©1992 National Academy of Sciences. Courtesy of National Academy Press, Washington DC

Box 6.2: Factors influencing the successful introduction of guidelines

Relative probability of being effective	*Development strategy*	*Dissemination strategy*	*Implementation strategy*
High	Internal	Specific educational intervention	Patient-specific reminder at time of consultation
Above average	Intermediate	Continuing medical education	Patient-specific feedback
Below average	External local	Posting targeted groups	General feedback
Low	External national	Publication in professional journal	General reminder of guidelines

Source: Grimshaw J M and Russell I T (1994) Achieving health gain through clinical guidelines. II Ensuring that guidelines change medical practice. *Quality in Health Care*, **3**:45–52.

elsewhere.[10] The figure shows that to improve quality one needs a vision, or a strategy, which must be based on the practice's needs but especially on patients' needs. Implementing that strategy depends on the practice culture – including leadership, teamworking, and communication – and on certain techniques, of which audit is one. Audit is important but, as shown in Figure 6.2, it is now included where it should be, as one of many techniques necessary for the provision of quality care.

Many TQM benefits can be derived by applying methods that have been used for many years, but in a co-ordinated way. Strategic planning is done in the context in which the strategy will be implemented; management systems are required for organising the practice; communication and teamwork skills are essential to the process; and audit is employed to identify problems and evaluate change.

The method can work, but even with this degree of multifaceted intervention there are deficiencies that need to be improved.[13] There is no incentive for practices to improve quality; education, so essential to all improvement, remains apart from quality improvement implementation; support for primary healthcare team development

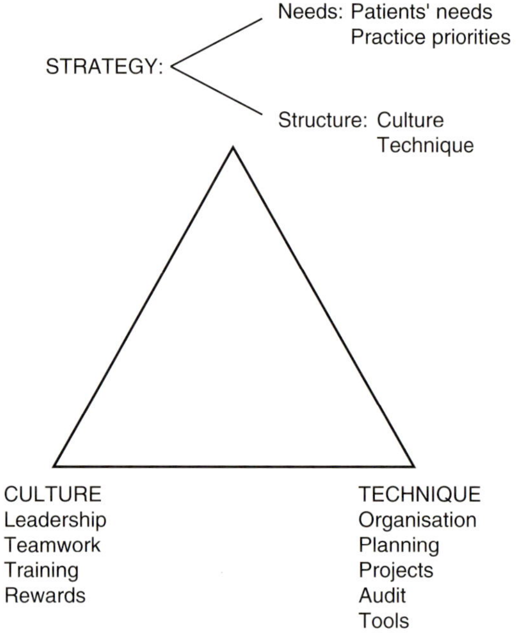

Figure 6.2: A framework for quality improvement in primary care.

is still split between the professions; and all such support has been given less priority by health authorities since family health service authorities have been incorporated into district health authorities.

Conclusion

Quality of primary care has improved enormously over the past 25 years. Not only have the best practices got better, but the generality of practices has improved overall. However, we have far to go, and at the same time primary healthcare itself is changing.

Patients are becoming better informed. The electronic data to which doctors began to have access about ten years ago are now available to patients and journalists. Patients are more demanding of healthcare, and see the need for access to a wider range of professionals than the GP on a one-to-one consultation. Primary healthcare will take place in a wider range of locations with a wider range of professionals.

Multiprofessional care will become the norm. Not only do GPs not have the skills to deal with all aspects of care, they do not have the time to handle all current demands. Primary healthcare must be seen as a multifocus, multiprovider system – and must be planned that way.

Paradoxically, this is exacerbated by patients being healthier. As the burden of severe disease recedes, there is greater incentive to consult for matters that relate to improving health and well-being, as well as screening for early disease. This requires a different form of primary care – an understanding of epidemiology, skill in a wide area of medical conditions, systematic practice protocols, and the deployment of a wide range of professionals in the primary healthcare team. It is the quality of the system that must be maintained, not only that of the individual practitioner.

Moreover, as health improves it is the community we must consider, not just practice populations. The government White Paper *The new NHS: modern, dependable* (December 1997) emphasises this by establishing primary care groups in which GPs and community services will work together, co-operating with social services, to improve the health of a population of around 100 000 people. Using quality improvement methodology, we should be able to work together with common aims, encouraging common systems and evaluating or monitoring using common criteria. But achieving such agreement will not be straightforward.

Implications for practice

The greatest emphasis must be to pool all our efforts. The stakeholders in different areas of quality improvement should co-ordinate their efforts since, however laudable it is to 'let many flowers grow', in the end co-ordination and organisation are required to produce a beautiful garden.

Perhaps most crucial is the integration of continuing education with service quality improvement. As demonstrated, the education and quality improvement movements have largely developed separately. However, most change only occurs if many influences, not just one, are applied and in particular 'education providers should develop multifaceted strategies, integrating their activities into the broad range of factors affecting change in practices'.[12] Moreover, many change projects that did not have educational input would have benefited if this component had been present.[12]

Not only are different aspects of medical care separated between service and education, but the education of various disciplines tends to be separate. This sets a pattern for separate professional development which becomes prolonged into mature working life. Practice nurses, managers, and health visitors all continue to go to their separate courses, which usually have no facilities for combining efforts. Primary healthcare team members get their education in very different arenas, and are then expected to work together with other disciplines.

Finally, primary care groups and health authorities have an important role to play in practice quality development. They have considerable financial power in supporting and giving direction to quality improvement. There is a strong public health imperative to focus on communities, assess broad needs, and commission secondary care. It is essential that primary care and public health work together in these areas. But we must remember that most healthcare takes place at the patient interface with primary care, and fostering quality improvement in the primary healthcare teams themselves is probably the most important factor of all in meeting patients' needs.

We have the tools: standard setting, performance evaluation, guidelines, audit, continuing education, a multidisciplinary team. We have developed many of these tools to a high level of sophistication. But the challenge of the next ten years is to integrate, coordinating theory and action, education and intervention, doctors and staff.

Summary

- Quality improvement initiatives, largely promoted by the RCGP, have had a major impact on primary healthcare over the past 25 years
- Development and assessment of vocational training practices have provided the most effective examples
- Audit is but one part of quality improvement, and its effectiveness has been impaired by its separation from continuing education
- Broader quality improvement methodologies, such as total quality management (TQM), are required for successful implementation of improvements in practice
- New structures in which quality improvement and continuing education groups work together, and in which disciplines co-operate, may again succeed in improving primary healthcare, especially in the new context of primary care groups responsible for whole communities

References

1 Pendleton D, Schofield T and Marinker M (eds) (1986) *In pursuit of quality*. Royal College of General Practitioners, London.
A collection of essays on quality, with comments by Avedis Donabedian. Two of the chapters are on the *New College course* and *What sort of doctor?*

2 Fleming D M and Lawrence M S (1993) The impact of audit on preventive measures. *British Medical Journal*, **287**:1852–4.
An early paper demonstrating the effect of audit and feedback.

3 Hasler J C and Schofield T P C (eds) (1984) *Continuing care in general practice*. Oxford University Press.
A succinct yet comprehensive guide to managing chronic disease in primary care.

4 Royal College of General Practitioners (1983) The quality initiative. *Journal of the Royal College of General Practitioners*, **33**:523–4.

5 Royal College of General Practitioners (1985) *What sort of doctor?* Report from general practice 23. RCGP, London.
A detailed report including assessment criteria, implementation methods and evaluation.

6 Schofield T P C and Hasler J C (1984) Approval of trainers and training practices in the Oxford Region. *British Medical Journal*, **288**:688–9.
A report of methods used for establishing and monitoring quality criteria for training.

7 Lawrence M S and Schofield T P C (eds) (1993) *Medical audit in primary health care*. Oxford University Press.
A book providing a comprehensive review of the theory and practice of audit.

8 Royal College of General Practitioners Clinical Guidelines Working Group (1995) *The development and implementation of guidelines in general practice*. Report from general practice 26. RCGP, London.
An overall review of the issues in guidelines for general practice.

9 The North of England Study of Standards and Performance in General Practice (1992) Medical audit in general practice I: Effects on doctors' clinical behaviour for common childhood conditions. *British Medical Journal*, **304**: 1480–4.
An example of the effect of guideline development in practice.

10 Pendleton D A and Hasler J C (1997) *Professional development in general practice*. Oxford University Press.
Chapter 9 considers the relationship of professional development and quality improvement – in particular summarising the nature and benefit of TQM (total quality management).

11 Davis D A, Thomson M A, Oxman A D and Haynes R B (1992) Evidence for the effectiveness of CME: a review of 50 randomised controlled trials. *Journal of the American Medical Association*, **268**:1111–17.

12 Allery L A, Owen P A and Robling M R (1997) Why general practitioners and consultants change their clinical practice: a critical incident study. *British Medical Journal*, **314**:870–4.
The above two papers consider the place and the effectiveness of education in improving service quality.

13 Lawrence M and Packwood T (1996) Adapting Total Quality Management for general practice: evaluation of a programme. *Quality in Health Care*, **5**:151–18.
A paper describing the effect of implementing a TQM programme in practice.

7

Understanding our discipline: the growth of informatics

Mike Pringle

Outline

- *The development of computers in general practice and their role in informatics*
  When computers first appeared, the interest was in the technology. Now the interest lies in their performance in supporting general practices to improve patient care
- *Informatics in the care of individual patients*
  Through both administrative and clinical roles, our information systems are offering a way to understand the clinical needs of individual patients for proactive and reactive care
- *Using informatics to understand and care for our practice populations*
  Health needs assessment and commissioning, on the foundation of intelligence derived from our databases, offers a route to improved healthcare services. The key role of primary care informatics in this process is explored
- *Professional development, and the way in which it can be facilitated by information*
  Our responsibility to develop ourselves and each other can be enhanced through the greater understanding of our educational needs that comes with high quality information

Introduction

Of course, every general practitioner wishes to do the best for his or her patients – apply up-to-date clinical knowledge tailored to the local context, with the accurate and effective use of interventions. The 'of course' is, of course, ironic: many general practitioners do not regard keeping up-to-date as a voyage of self-improvement but a point-accumulating chore; most do not understand their local context; evidence is often not available on the effectiveness of interventions; and accuracy is all too often left to chance.

It is these issues that informatics is set to address, and this chapter will reflect on the promise that computers, through their outputs rather than their structures or processes, can deliver. First, however, the development of primary care informatics is discussed.

The development of primary care informatics

Although the term 'informatics' is usually associated with computers, computers are only a tool in the pursuit of the goals of information handling. Those practices involved in the early years of vocational training discovered the emphasis put on good medical records – in the author's training practice in Sonning Common they had achieved semi-religious status – and on registers. Although hospital records continued to be unmanageable and incoherent and the Lloyd George envelope developed dark mystic corners within its barely suppressed anarchy, records made on A4-sized paper were designed to make a patient's story accessible to a doctor.

Although these A4 records were not a requirement for good care, they marked a cultural turning point in which 'a doctor's *aide-mémoire*' became a tool for co-ordinated team care. This new culture gave the clinical record a respect, an accuracy and a functionality that it had previously lacked. With problem lists and immunisation sheets, antenatal records, pathology reports, and legible and semi-legible continuation records, these records set out the template for the development of computer records.

It is difficult to pinpoint the first attempts at using computers in primary care, but the laurels probably go to Michael Abrams who reported crude computerised recall systems as early as 1968. In the 1970s, the Exeter Community Health Services Computer Project was using a central mainframe and practice-based terminals – a similar configuration to that used in the Oxford Region in the mid 1970s.

This Oxford scheme, led by John Perry, involved a network of practices linked by a landline to the mainframe in Oxford. Each practice, including Sonning Common, had a single terminal into which a limited range of data was entered. An age-sex register, immunisation and cervical cytology recalls, and major problems (coded in OXMIS) were stored centrally and printouts were delivered back to the practices.

While the landline was painfully slow and the breakdowns numerous, the printouts were crude, and the ergonomic advantages over a card index in a shoebox hard to define, the essence of modern and future informatics were present in this pilot scheme. There was a culture that valued information for a patient-based and a population approach to general practice, and partners willing to explore systems for improving that information.

By the late 1970s, microcomputers were being introduced and the prospect of widespread, if ruinously expensive, practice-based computers began to be discussed. A report by a working party of the Royal College of General Practitioners, *Computers in primary care*, was published in 1980, and for many involved in informatics this offered, for the first time, a functional framework within which we could envisage the development of a new generation of information systems. In particular, the authors tried to hold back the tide of 'techydom' in which the boxes are more important that the product: 'The development of general practice computer systems and the parallel development of clinical standards to which the whole profession is already committed are closely inter-related'.

Unfortunately 'techydom' won. In the 'Micros for general practitioners scheme' in 1982, 140 practices – of the 1015 that applied – were offered heavily subsidised computers. Considering that it was estimated that only 50 practices had a computer at that time, this was a remarkable investment; but it was founded on the great illusion that a computer, of itself, solves problems. The programs were so poor and the functionality so limited that these systems offered no real benefits to patient care.

This was also the era of the home-made system, some of which survive today. General practitioners would buy a crude computer with dual floppy disc drives and a simple programming language, and set about reinventing the wheel. While it is an excellent training in logic and computer science, these early efforts were seldom given the development support needed to make them generalisable. The few that were became the next generation of GP systems which took advantage of the personal computer (PC) era when it brought cheaper, faster computers within the financial reach of most practices.

By the end of the 1980s, technology still ruled informatics. There were assumptions in health service management that the 'level of computerisation' in an area was an indicator of quality. Any practice worth its salt had to have a computer in the corner, if only to generate repeat prescriptions. The recurrent surveys of GP computerisation undertaken by the Department of Health showed increasing installation of computers and increasing numbers of functions being computerised. However, the reality was that most computers were being used for a limited range of unimaginative tasks – recalls, repeat prescribing – and their real potential had yet to be exploited.

One crucial innovation was the Read codes devised by James Read to develop a comprehensive coded clinical thesaurus. True, there were many coding systems in place before and several more since – ICD, OXMIS, ICHPPC, RCGP and more recently ICPC – but these were either unstructured or were geared to the generation of aggregate data. None was useful for coding the clinical record as a structured alternative to the manual record in the care of a patient. When James Read started gathering clinical codes together into his original thesaurus he could not have anticipated the dramatic pace of their adoption, nor some of the problems that changes in computer use and international classification might bring. However, his work underpins the potential for informatics that this chapter will discuss.

There was much that was seen to be wrong about the NHS reforms in the late 1980s and early 1990s, not least the manner of their imposition, but they focused minds wonderfully on the way in which technology could be applied. Through three key elements – targets, medical audit and fundholding – the reforms stimulated thinking along two parallel, but interconnected, lines: clinical and managerial.

In the surveys of GP computerisation many practices had reported consultation use of their computers, but in effect this meant checking a few details and issuing prescriptions. The real functions were still administrative, although most of these were linked to the patient record. In most practices the manual record still ruled supreme in the care of individual patients. As the medico-legal and technical dimensions of a computer clinical record became clearer, however, the manual record became increasingly subordinate to the computer record. In the 1990s, the arrival of the electronic health record (EHR) in practices throughout Britain can be proclaimed.

This is not to say that the computers' administrative role decreased. In fundholding, of course, the transactions of care, especially referrals, had to be entered and monitored; for target payments and health promotion banding, preventive care needed to be accurately recorded. At last practices had a reason to ask for and record lifestyle details and the computer record began to contain a depth and accuracy of data to which, historically, few manual systems aspired.

Medical audit was, of course, welcomed by everybody as the only part of the reform package which was unequivocally positive – almost certainly because nobody truly understood to what they were signing up. However, in many practices the imperative to start auditing offered the first real justification for the entry of high quality clinical data onto their computers. Their disease registers were being used for more than the care of individual patients; the accuracy of a diagnostic entry for asthma, diabetes or ischaemic heart disease became important.

However, in the second half of the 1990s, the dialogue has changed, thankfully, away from the technology to the outcomes, the benefits for patient care. The techies, with their EPROMs and their CPUs, have been routed. Now, it is possible to visualise the ways in which practice databases help in offering better patient care – in other words, informatics.

What does informatics offer general practice?

This section will describe how informatics is revolutionising care for individual patients and populations. However, it also has significant implications for practices as organisations and for the personal and professional development of GPs themselves.

All GPs are used to being surrounded by data. The manual records contain mountains of them and they are bombarded by new 'facts' in journals, books, newspapers, and on television. Additionally, they have access to their own experience and the experience of other clinicians in their practices (doctors and nurses), colleagues in other practices and hospital doctors, a depth of wisdom that is too rarely tapped. Historically, the importance of 'wisdom' was that some people, through thought and experience, were able to make sense of the wealth of data in the environment and offer guidance that seemed to the recipient to have credibility. The same applies today to medical wisdom, and it is a precious resource that must not be ignored in the rush to exploit computer-based informatics.

Although GPs must continue to read editorials and to share their experience with colleagues, they will increasingly have another source for reference. The forte of a computer is to turn data into information. In other words, it prepares data for assimilation by the human brain. That is not, however, the end of the story. Information must be turned into knowledge (a process that requires the integration of experience, evidence and information from other sources). Knowledge then must be turned into behavioural change (and we all know how difficult that is!). And finally that change in behaviour must, in the context of primary care, be shown to improve patient care, individually or collectively (*see* Figure 7.1).

This is a tall order, and it can be seen immediately that the role of a computerised information system is small compared to the role of the human being. It is ourselves who must arrive at the knowledge that informs our decisions, it is us who must change our behaviour, and it is us who are responsible to our patients for the quality of their care. Our information systems can facilitate us, no more, in this evolution of quality, and this section will illustrate some ways in which that might occur.

Informatics in the care of individual patients

The consultation, with its medical and social interchange between patient and GP, is central to our discipline. While the essentials of high level communication within an ethical framework of respect and mutual endeavour will remain largely untainted by informatics,

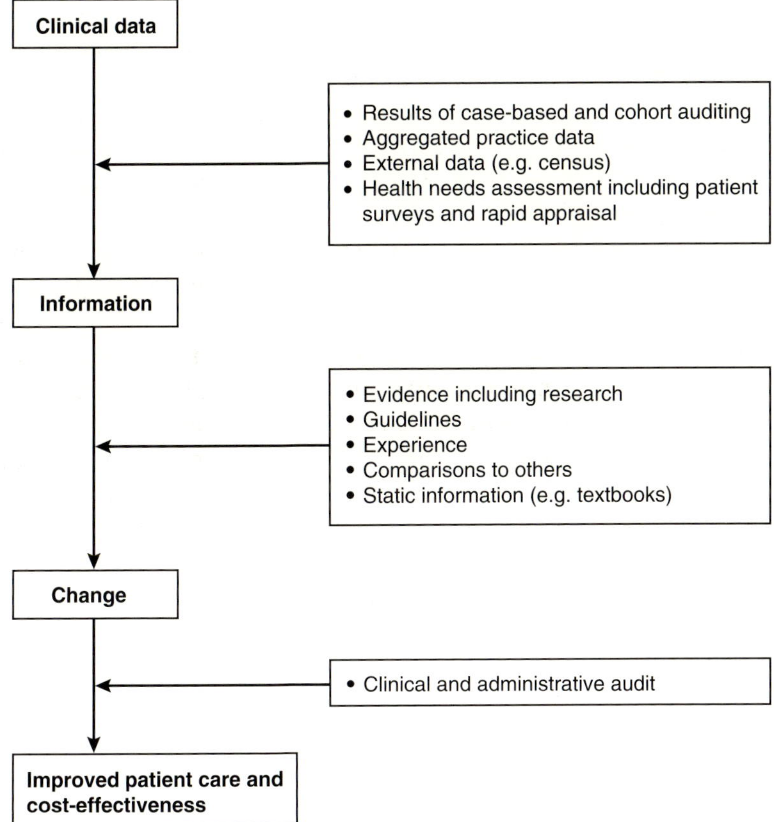

Figure 7.1: The contribution of informatics to quality improvement in general practice.

these are not the only essentials of a successful consultation. Often undervalued is the underlying assumption of clinical competency: the right diagnosis and the right management plan.

Already, computer systems offer us a patient's record in more flexible formats than could be possible from the traditional manual record. The doctor can look at key problems, or all reasons for encounters; can look at consultations chronologically or by problem; can check on risk factors as a separate screen or window, as flashing reminders or as an integrated part of the clinical record.

Increasingly, the use of graphics will speed the GP's ability to assimilate data as information: a graph of hypertensive control and creatinine levels may highlight a trend towards deteriorating renal function associated with inadequate hypertensive control, and do so much more immediately and eloquently than any fragmented clinical record. The human brain's capacity to absorb images rather than text has, so far, hardly been exploited by our information systems.

Delivering a patient's record into our consciousness may be a considerable aid for quality of care to that individual, but if that were the sole justification for the investment of our time, money and emotion, the case for computerisation would be thin. However, already our computer systems are improving our decision-making in many ways – some small, some substantial.

We are all familiar with the 'reminders' that appear at some point as we enter a patient's record. We are told that the prescription file needs renewing, that a cervical smear is due, that a review of hypertension should have occurred in January. Many prefer to leave these doctor-centred aspects towards the end of the consultation unless they relate to the reason for the patient's decision to consult. However, these reminders presage the potential for reinforced routine actions. They are all the more powerful when they are context-specific, such as reminders of penicillin allergy when prescribing an antibiotic.

When a diagnosis or problem title is selected for an encounter, the possibility of reminders of specific data entry and diagnosis-related activities arises. Many practices have protocols, often derived from national or local guidelines, that all clinicians – nurses and doctors – have signed up to as a team. Whenever these protocols can be linked to a disease or procedure code, a template is generated that acts as a reminder and mentor.

For example, if *hyperlipidaemia* is selected from a patient's problem list as the reason for an encounter, a template might remind the GP about those data items and actions that the practice team agreed would accompany the care of such patients. First, the doctor might check that the latest fasting total cholesterol, HDL, LDL and triglycerides have been entered correctly. Then a reminder confirms whether a blood sugar, TSH, CK, and LFTs have been entered within the past two years and, if not recently updated, the patient's smoking and alcohol consumption can be entered. The GP can insert details of the patient's family history as well as symptoms, such as angina and breathlessness. The opportunity to enter a blood pressure and weight is given and the BMI is calculated using a previous height entry.

The template can then move into the area of decision support. It can remind the clinician if lipid control is inadequate and can prompt questions concerning management. Has diet been discussed? If appropriate, has treatment with lipid-lowering drugs been considered? If so, has the right drug been chosen in the right dose? Have side-effects been asked for? If treatment was discontinued, was it because of undesired effects?

In this way, the computer's software becomes a sophisticated reminder of actions specifically relevant to an individual patient. Another example of this is Prodigy, a program that is designed to facilitate more cost-effective prescribing. It links management advice to specific Read codes and will offer a quick route into a number of prescriptions for many conditions, advising simple management and then cheaper medication when it is likely to be effective.

Prodigy also offers a shortcut into patient information. As an adjunct to an explanation to the patient, the program can be asked to print out a summary of key points of information for the patient, usually on the blank paper beside the prescription, to act as an *aide-mémoire.* Not only can such information be more easily available than rummaging in drawers for a leaflet received several years ago, but it can be personalised to incorporate the messages that are most relevant to that patient. All such decision supports can be overridden – indeed, must be overridden – when the circumstances of a patient requires it; they are there to help, not to dictate.

In time, we will be able to access more sophisticated information which can help to inform our decision-making with individual cases. For example, information concerning our performance in a clinical area will be fed back to us at the point at which decisions are taken that would influence our decisions.

To continue with the example of the patient with hyperlipidaemia, soon doctors will be able to see how they are doing in comparison to the criteria and standards of care to which they have signed up. They will compare their care for an individual patient to their average achievement of the criteria for patients with hyperlipidaemia seen by themselves, partners or teams in other practices. Supposing that a doctor has agreed that the treatment objective should be that patients with hypercholesterolaemia should have serum cholesterols under 6.5 mg/100 ml, to be achieved in 80% of cases.

The patient being reviewed has a cholesterol of 6.8 mg/100 ml and the doctor is reminded of the agreed standard of care. Then the doctor is given the current (and continuously updated) results of his or her own and the practice's success in moving towards the criteria and agreed standards, and how other doctors who contribute to a data-sharing network are doing. Having access to information about how we compare to ourselves in the past, our expectations and the normative behaviour of those in the practice and elsewhere – interactive audit – offers considerable potential for turning information into knowledge and thus into behavioural change.

Another form of information to enhance the care of individual patients comes from outside the practice. In its simplest form it can substitute for MIMS and BNF by offering ready access to simple repetitive facts such as dosages, contraindications, side-effects, interactions, etc. Access to on-line medical textbooks can allow a GP to consult an information source to establish or check facts relevant to a particular patient. More exciting, perhaps, is the possibility of access to evidence that is more relevant to the specific patient than the generic information from reference books. Has a rash ever been reported from this particular drug in a female patient in her thirties? How unusual is a diagnosis of migraine in the elderly and has it been associated with the onset of diabetes as appears to be the case with this patient?

Some of these questions can be answered by aggregated databases from practices; some will require interested GPs to value and share their collective knowledge and understanding, the wisdom referred to earlier, probably through electronic networks. Whatever the mechanism, it seems likely that we will, in time, be formulating questions which now we would regard as fanciful – and we will expect meaningful answers.

Informatics in the care of our patient populations

Already we know far more about our patient population than we might have dreamt possible a decade ago. Many can recall the excitement of a first age-sex bar chart, a table of the practice population by postcode, or a validated count of patients with diabetes. Those small victories should not be decried; these were the early days of trying to make the technology produce something that the practice could use to plan its care.

General practice computer systems open up the possibility of readily turning data into information. The generation of, for example, uptake rates for cervical cytology and childhood immunisations is taken for granted. Many practices know, month by month, the rate of recording of lifestyle factors such as smoking and alcohol, risk factors like weight, blood pressure, family history or cholesterol, the prevalence of chronic diseases and the incidence of acute diagnoses, workload and work rates, referral and investigation rates, and prescribing information. These items of information, derived almost exclusively from a practice database, help a primary healthcare team to understand their business – the business of delivering healthcare to their registered list.

There are two dimensions that need adding to this routine level of data aggregation to make it come alive. The first is quality assurance and the other is external data; between them these all add up to health needs assessment.

Some practices hold regular 'significant event' meetings. At these, clinical events which have occurred in the past month are discussed. These might include all acute myocardial infarctions, strokes, attempted or successful suicides; serious infections such as meningitis; acute visits or admissions for diabetes, asthma, or epilepsy; positive cervical smear or case of whooping cough; and every patient complaint, administrative failure (such as a visit accepted but not done) or prescribing error. Although some significant events are noted by a team member and some are spotted in hospital discharge letters, the list of events can also be derived from computer entries.

Traditional auditing involves the examination of aggregated patient data against agreed criteria and standards. Almost all of such data can be derived from a computerised database.

Since hyperlipidaemia seems to have developed as a theme of this chapter, the role of computerised audit will be illustrated through a man with high blood fats. About two years ago a patient of mine, a popular local builder, died from a sudden myocardial infarction. He was 52 years old. At the significant event discussion it emerged that for eight years I had been treating his hypercholesterolaemia with a diet and for six years essential hypertension with medication. He was a lean, fit, non-smoker whose father died of a coronary in his early fifties. I knew therefore about his risks and I had been trying to minimise the ones that were amenable to change. So far so good, and my partners were quick to congratulate me. This, incidentally, is a key benefit of significant event auditing – good practice is identified as well as the less good.

In our discussions we all acknowledged a sense of unease over our management of raised cholesterol. We had been loath to lurch into active management beyond dietary advice, but recent trials and editorials had suggested a more aggressive approach would be justified. As a result of these discussions we undertook an audit and found that we had only 29 patients with a diagnosis of hyperlipidaemia and only 65 patients had a cholesterol level entered onto the computer.

Thus, a significant event had led us to ask a conventional audit question and the computer had supplied the data for us to start to expand our understanding. At this point we understood that we had a problem, but not what we ought to do about it. We also needed to put this problem alongside all the others we were facing and to prioritise it.

Routine data collection helps to define the topography, but clinical audit, often by the nature of the way in which the question is derived, offers texture to that topography. In order to derive a full health needs assessment a practice needs to appreciate the views of the community, as expressed through patient surveys and rapid appraisal, and externally collected data such as from the census, general household surveys, lifestyle surveys and so on.

Using such varied sources of information a practice team can derive a rounded picture of the health of its population and establish the extent to which the practice is 'normal' in experiencing traditional needs (perhaps the average rate of total hip replacement), or unusual in having special requirements (e.g. a high rate of teenage pregnancy). And then there is the important element of team preference. Faced with a range of identified health needs, a practice must quantify and then value each, deciding what must be done and what should be done to offer the highest quality cost-effective care to the registered list.

In this case, we decided that the management of raised lipids would be a priority for us. So our task was then to convert this case-derived information into knowledge and thus into improved care. For this we needed to know the results of research from the published literature and any available guidelines; this needed to be interpreted in the light of our own experience and that of others. We consulted a clinical biochemist and two cardiologists.

As a team, we then established a protocol for the practice that identified high risk people for a high level of intervention: those with ischaemic heart disease, hypertension or diabetes with a fasting cholesterol over 6.5 mg/100 ml. We agreed to try diet first but, if not wholly successful, to move quickly to medication after confirmation that the creatine kinase, random blood sugar, TSH and liver function tests were normal. In order to make these decisions stick we developed a template and audited our care every three months. We also agreed an allocation of £50k from our fundholding budget to pay for this increase in service.

Two years later we had 384 patients with a diagnosis of hyperlipidaemia – a 13-fold increase. Of these, 80% have had a lipid profile recorded within the past 14 months, although 99% have in fact consulted in that period. For 19% of these patients their last serum cholesterol was over 7.5 mg/100 ml; 27% were between 6.5 and 7.5; and over half, 54%, were under our target of 6.5 mg/100 ml.

While being far from satisfied with this performance, it does represent a considerable move from the state of inertia of two years before. It demonstrates the power of databases to offer insights, to aid the accumulation and interpretation of new knowledge and, through commissioning and feedback, to ensure that improvements in care are not just agreed but do occur.

Informatics in the development of the practice

A key benefit from the advent of the computer into the consultation, all consultations by all clinicians in the practice, has been an increase in understanding about each other. The doctors understand which patients choose which doctor through differences in the characteristics of caseloads. One partner may see more of the elderly, while another sees more psychological medicine. A female partner, predictably but perhaps regrettably, may attract gynaecological problems and contraception.

In significant event discussions and through clinical auditing, but especially in protocol development meetings, all team members can share their clinical knowledge and constructs. Practice nurses offer an important dimension to these discussions. In understanding which patients consult them and in learning from them about their experience and knowledge base, a team can build a cohesive view of its clinical task. The practice manager can add an understanding of the commissioning process and resource usage to inform discussions.

It is this shared understanding based on collective experience and a common knowledge about patients, priorities and aspirations, and the progress that is being made towards shared goals, that links informatics to practice development. As a tool for joint learning and development, it is unparalleled.

Informatics in the personal and professional development of GPs

So it comes back to us as individual practitioners, and how informatics can help us grow. Inevitably we grow as clinicians through using informatics to improve our patients' care, both as individuals and collectively, and inevitably we grow as informatics helps us to build our teams. However, personal development demands more than that. It demands that we develop insight into our strengths and weaknesses, and that we exploit our strengths and address our weaknesses. The defining of educational needs can be facilitated through the use of information systems; differences from other practitioners can be highlighted and repetitive quirks defined.

A GP might, for example, see that she tolerates poorer control in hypertension than do her partners. She might be using a wider range of drugs for treating hypertension and some of these might be in lower doses than is usual for her partners. From this she might conclude that she needs to brush up on the management of hypertension. This might be through reading review articles or textbooks. She might hold a seminar in the practice and learn from her colleagues. Alternatively, she might attend a lecture, go on a course, or find a distance-learning package. After she has been educated and has had an opportunity to put her new understanding into practice, the information system can help her to demonstrate improved care for hypertension. The role of informatics in continuing professional development may be profound.

Another way in which doctors can develop is through matching themselves against generally accepted definitions of high quality care. At the onset of their careers, GPs undertake summative assessment and the Membership of the RCGP, and later they can do Membership by Assessment of Performance. Since 1989, Fellowship by Assessment of the RCGP has offered a way to demonstrate the highest standards, and for this a candidate must show that all 60 criteria are met. Not surprisingly, many of these require information about the practice through significant event auditing, clinical auditing, workload analysis, resource usage and preventive care levels. And a GP with good information systems has the foundation on which to build an application for Membership by Assessment of Performance, or Fellowship by Assessment.

General practitioners, practice nurses, community nurses and practice managers are increasingly becoming involved in research. While computer databases can seldom, alone, answer our research questions they offer an excellent tool for hypothesis generation, piloting and patient sampling. Those GPs who are not yet ready for the full plunge into research might prefer to share in aggregated databases which others can use for research. The number of research collaborators is growing every year, and each is gaining an incentive to improve their database in order to contribute to the research endeavour in the medical community.

Conclusion

The move away from a fascination with technology towards what information can provide for clinicians, practices, and individuals has been important for general practice. Informatics holds out the promise of incremental improvements in the quality of care and of personal development within practices. That is not an inconsequential claim.

Most importantly, informatics offers access to that most precious of all commodities – wisdom. Wisdom to understand patients; wisdom to see how their care can be improved; wisdom to develop teams; and wisdom in personal growth. It was the application of wisdom that inspired me as a vocational trainee in Sonning Common, and it is the pursuit of excellence through wisdom to which I aspire now in my professional practice.

Summary

- The informatics flow, the turning of data into improved patient care, has always been available: the new dimension is the GP's capacity to use computerised databases to allow improvement of efficiency with which data are linked to quality
- As interest has moved from the technology towards its function, a new range of skills and abilities has been developed. These offer exciting possibilities for individual patients, the practice population and the GP's personal development
- Enhanced information in the consultation, including relevant reminders, some decision support and interactive clinical audit, allows a better understanding of individual patients and their care
- Knowing more about the population of registered patients allows a more effective use of resources and care planning in the context of health needs
- Having greater insight into ourselves, as GPs, our strengths and weaknesses, allows us to plan our education and personal development effectively and to monitor its effect

Further reading

Marinker M (ed) (1990) *Medical audit and general practice.* British Medical Journal Publications, London.

Pringle M, Bradley C, Carmichael C, Wallis H and Moore A (1995) *Significant event auditing.* Occasional Paper 70. RCGP, London.

Pringle M, Hayden J and Procter A (1996) *A guide for new principals.* Oxford University Press, London.

Royal College of General Practitioners (1990) *Fellowship by assessment.* Occasional paper 50. RCGP, London. (2e 1996)

Royal College of General Practitioners (1995) *The development and implementation of clinical guidelines.* RCGP, London.

8

Evaluating practice: developing relevant research capacity

Ann-Louise Kinmonth

Outline

This chapter argues the need to develop the research wing of general practice in ways that respect the particular nature of general practice. This will involve recognition of the importance of the perspective of each individual in their social context as well as evidence from the population perspectives of epidemiology, and the cellular perspectives of the laboratory.

A review of the changing organisation of practice, including the rise of team care and focus on prevention, makes the case for research spanning both organisation of care and its delivery within the consultation. A review of academic general practice makes the case for increasing research capacity through the development of both clinical academic careers, and inclusion of a range of non-clinical disciplines, and the use of both quantitative and qualitative research methods.

Finally, examples are given from the author's experience of a multidisciplinary approach to research in general practice, and parallels are drawn between the strengths of the team approach to both practice and research.

Introduction

Good general medical practice values the specific experience and social situation of the individual as well as general knowledge of the natural history of disease and its treatment. Pressure is now rising to base practice on evidence, rather than experience, and to offer 'team' care to populations rather than simply personal medical care to individuals.

If academic general practice is to assist practitioners in reconciling these tensions, it must develop a methodological approach to research that respects the particular nature of general practice. This will involve developing strong collaborations with the social and behavioural sciences as well as the traditional biological disciplines.

This collaboration is necessary if the questions we ask and the answers we find are to relate to the whole person, so making sense to every doctor, and to be incorporated most easily into daily practice.

The tradition of individual care

A young doctor contemplating a career in general medical practice at the end of the 20th century is inheriting a fine tradition of the medical care of individuals in the context of their social lives. The general practitioner bridges not only generalist and specialist care, but also the consultation between the experience of illness and the abstraction of disease; helping to make sense of the causes of symptoms and the interaction between person and environment, often mediated by behaviour. This tradition is well summarised in the 15th century epithet; '*guérir quelquefois, soulager souvent, consoler toujours*' quoted by Sir Theodore Fox in his Harveian oration of 1965.[1] In this essay on the purposes of medicine, Fox argues that the doctor's overriding duty is to the individual:

> … his duty is to treat his neighbour as himself, and this task is at once natural and sophisticated, simple and exacting – for no two people are alike; and each can change from hour to hour. Not least do people differ in their attitude to life – some cling to it as a miser to his money and to as little purpose. Others wear it lightly, ready to risk it for a cause, a hope, a song, the wind in their face.

As Ian McWhinney argues so persuasively, general practice defines itself in terms of the relationship between doctor and patient, and above all, each patient wants to be recognised, appreciated and understood. Doctors busy 'doing to' patients risk losing their capacity to recognise suffering. Iona Heath, in her elegant John Fry Trust Monograph, describes the doctor as 'witness and companion to the patient's journey'.[2] McWhinney maintains that if our clinical method does not have this recognition, with witness at its centre, it will fail at its deepest level, and we will have lost our capacity and privilege to comfort always.[3]

How is the young doctor to make sense of this tradition of commitment to the individual in the face of the changing nature of medicine?

The rise of team care for populations

The old ideal of the personal physician, responding as part of the community to the needs of the individuals within it, as epitomised by Dr Lydgate in George Eliot's *Middlemarch*, seems at odds with the new paradigm of team healthcare for registered populations. In a scant hundred years we have moved from the pre-antibiotic era, where the individual doctor could do little more than be a sympathetic witness to events, to the deployment of a range of powerful medications and treatments via the primary healthcare team (PHCT), which is increasingly involved in purchasing and providing comprehensive primary care for registered populations.

Paradoxically, despite their improved social circumstances, individuals within these populations are making ever more demands on the ever larger PHCT. The national morbidity statistics for general practice show that consulting rates in UK general practice have risen over the last ten years across almost the whole range of classified symptoms. Similarly, the National Association for the Welfare of Children in Hospital reports that a preschool child has a greater chance of admission to hospital today than at any time in the past. People's expectations of medical care seem to be rising and their tolerance of discomfort and uncertainty falling.

Expectations of cure are fuelled by palpable medical advances and yet, in the midst of this optimism, it is still true that the prevalent chronic disorders and cancers of our ageing society can often only be ameliorated. And as specialist care in hospitals becomes ever more technical, it seems that the clinical skills of amelioration are being seen more and more as the province of continuing care in general practice.

Preventive medicine

Increasing technical ability and rising expectation, in combination with a shift of responsibility from specialist to generalist care, have resulted in a rising workload in general practice. This is exacerbated further by the institution of systematic preventive medicine; for GPs now have explicit responsibility for the health of the populations registered with them. This responsibility was set out in the 1990 Contract between the National Health Service and GPs. It includes seeking out and managing individuals at risk of disease as well as responding to the symptoms and anxieties of those who consult.

In effect, GPs are now charged with finding those whose dice appear to be loaded against them and seeing what can be done to restore the balance. The costs and benefits for individuals of encumbering their personal doctors with this responsibility for the public health are still unclear to many doctors. Even those who are convinced are more comfortable with case funding among high risk groups than trying to shift the risk of society, as a whole, by screening populations.

The general practitioners' response

On the whole, practitioners are taking the steady rise in expectation and workload rather badly. The new recruit will see a range of responses; from dogged persistence or early retirement on the one hand, to new definitions of the job of the GP and its organisation, on the other. One such response has been the expansion and development of highly organised team care supported by increasingly sophisticated information technology.

This response was further stimulated by the previous Conservative government's policy of splitting the purchaser and provider roles in the NHS and encouraging GPs to take a lead voice in purchasing, alongside health authorities or in collaboration with them. Under these circumstances, practice management and nursing have both developed strongly; and there are many examples of such a team achieving both more appropriate and more comprehensive primary care, as described by John Hasler in his own John Fry Trust Monograph, *Teamwork in Primary Care.*

A Labour government replaced the Conservatives in spring 1997. It has produced White Papers on primary care, public health and the NHS during its first year of office which continue to fuel change.

Another response has been explicit delineation of the appropriate limits to the work of the generalist physician, often leading to the doctor focusing most strongly on the more technical aspects of medicine, the 'doing to' aspects, and defining the time and emotion involved in 'being with' patients as better done by nurses or a range of 'counsellors'. Another response has been simply to work ever harder at the expense of self and family. It is difficult to believe that the spectacle of these responses is not contributory to the serious drop in recruitment of young doctors to general practice.

Young physicians are highly vocationally committed (although quite rightly more assertive about the importance of a full life of which professional practice is but one, albeit important part). They want to know what the implications of the continuing changes in general practice are, both for the profession's underlying values, and for its contribution to relieving sickness and promoting health. It is a core responsibility of academic general practice to respond to this need. Together, the relevant academic branches of the discipline must provide evidence and education for students and doctors that will place them in a position to make the best choices about the organisation and delivery of care both within the practice as a whole and with each patient in the consultation. How is the academic wing of general practice progressing in this regard?

Academic general practice

All the clinical disciplines of medicine have an academic branch responsible for education, research, and much of the leadership of the profession. In the case of general practice, this academic branch has been a late development, strongly supported through the Royal College of General Practitioners (RCGP) which has provided an important academic focus campaigning for vocational training for general practice, and the establishment of university departments of general practice with their responsibility for undergraduate education, as well as for continuing professional development.

Links between the undergraduate and postgraduate academic divisions of general practice are now occurring, and the academic branch of general practice is suddenly flourishing – somewhat like a frontier town, full of excitement, inspiration and innovation. Similarly, the first professors of general practice were a bit like the early settlers, individualists with independent views and a capacity to survive isolation. For, until recently, academic general practice has been a very marginal activity, viewed slightly askance by practitioners on the one hand, and by colleagues in the medical school on the other.

From the medical school's perspective, general practice can seem too pragmatic, too applied, not confronting or answering any of the 'big' questions. Academic value in biomedicine is attached to a strong theoretical base, to understanding biological mechanisms, to causation, estimation and prediction. From this perspective, the highest value is attached to medicine as a branch of science where 'the pursuit of truth seems a higher adventure than the cure of Mrs Smith's ulcer' and where medical specialisation seems closer to the scientific paradigm, and so of higher value, than the apparent disorder of generalist practice.[1,4–6]

Many GPs themselves subscribe to this view at least partially, as a result of the attitudes and values absorbed at the specialists' knee during medical school training, evident in the fact that much continuing medical education for GPs is still provided (by the generalists' own choice) by specialists.

From this perspective, advances in practice 'trickle down' from the laboratory, through specialist practice to primary care; and professional development owes more to organised political action by practising colleagues than to abstract, 'ivory tower' research by general practice academics. This should not be too surprising since those now in practice have grown up in a branch of medicine which alone among the major clinical disciplines offered no academic career path and no recognition of the value of research within its contract of employment.

However, the changes in medical practice and society that have produced such tensions for the GP have stimulated a dramatic growth in the academic branch of the discipline. This stimulation has come both from the anticipated shift in teaching medical students from hospital to the community, where the patients are, and from the establishment of the research and development strategy for the NHS as a whole – with its focus on developing, for the first time, a specific knowledge base for general as well as specialist practice.

It is not that there was no tradition of general practice research in the past but that it was carried out by remarkable individuals informed by and informing their own clinical practice. (Thus, Mackenzie's *Principles of diagnosis and treatment in heart conditions* depended on careful observation of the natural history of heart disease in individuals cared for by him over many years; Pickles' observations of the spread of infection depended on his responsibility for a small isolated population and his close knowledge of the social contacts of individuals within it.) Rather, there had been no strong tradition of academic groups investigating particular topics and building up particular approaches to research in general practice.

There are now departments of general practice in all the medical schools in the UK, and the first professors of the subject in the oldest universities of Oxford and Cambridge are under election or have recently been elected. In some universities, GPs hold deanships in medical education, and general practice contributes significantly to new community-based curricula and to the final examinations.

However, academic general practice is still very small, both absolutely and relatively. Thus, when reviewed by the Richards Taskforce on clinical academic careers in 1997, there were about 335 members of the Association of University Departments of General Practice among 31 950 principals; compared with 2384 clinical academics (professors, readers, senior lecturers and lecturers) among 19 110 consultants in all the hospital specialities combined. This gives a ratio of clinical academics to principals of 0.01 compared with that of clinical academics to all consultants of 0.12.

There is a dearth of clinical academics in the discipline with appropriate training in research methods, as evidenced by the few GPs who take up national research training awards, and by the few who are ready to take on the responsibilities of heading the established departments of general practice, let alone the burgeoning postgraduate departments in the newer universities.

To some extent, academic general practice is in danger of being the casualty of its own success; drowning in the bow wave of the development of community-based education, and the demand for evidence-based practice. For in the scramble to satisfy the demands of others, there is a risk of losing sight of the core challenge facing research efforts in general practice. This challenge includes taking the time necessary to develop a methodological approach that respects the particular nature of general practice. Only if research methods value the specific experience of the individual, as well as general knowledge of the natural history of the disease and its treatment, will the knowledge that is uncovered be felt to be relevant by the young colleagues who look to academics for help.

Similarly, only if the questions asked make sense in the light of day-to-day practice will the answers be applied there. To get methods right involves drawing on the disciplines of the social and behavioural sciences, as well as those of the biomedical sciences; 'getting the questions right' involves immersion in general practice and confronting the uncertainties of the consulting room with a clear mind.

The disciplines underpinning general practice

There are many examples of physicians (generalist and specialist) collaborating with epidemiologists to advance the understanding of organ-based disease and its management. Many of the studies carried out through the Medical Research Council's general practice framework are of this nature; furthering understanding, for example, of hypertension, hypercoagulability, and ischaemic heart disease, and of their management. These studies combine population-based methods, studying the distributions of diseases and their causes in populations, with clinical and laboratory work. There is a great need for continuing denominator-based work of this kind at the level of the common presenting symptoms in general practice.

Such work goes beyond the 'trickle down' model of extrapolating evidence from studies on patients attending hospital in very important ways. It studies the natural history of symptoms such as headache, earache, sore throat, which are either rarely seen in specialist practice or, when they are, exhibit different patterns of underlying pathology and prognosis.

The costs and benefits of different investigative and therapeutic strategies depend crucially on the prevalence of serious pathology in the population studied; a course of action well justified by a high prevalence of underlying disease in hospital practice may be harmful and wasteful in primary care. However, to inform cost-effective care of individual patients in their social context, social and psychological epidemiology and health economics must be added to clinical epidemiology.

The GP wants to know the effects of management, not only on symptom resolution, but also on patients' anxiety, quality of life, well-being and satisfaction with management. He or she wants to know what effects the practitioner's behaviour may have on the attitude of the patient to his or her treatment and self-care; and while interested in the general truths about these issues at the population level, is most concerned about the best ways to adapt knowledge of the general successfully to the particulars presented by the individual patient.

Research on these issues depends on in-depth study of individual experiences of illness in specific social settings, as well as at population level. It draws on the skills of qualitative researchers, such as sociologists and anthropologists, its purpose being understanding and explanation, not prediction; it broadens and enriches the more quantitative work aimed at prediction and generalisability and, well used, can root research in the enduring ground of the consultation itself.

The rise of the multidisciplinary research team

This approach to research is leading to the development of multidisciplinary research teams, and involves statisticians, epidemiologists, health economists, psychologists, sociologists and others to work in collaboration with clinicians. Together, they are developing approaches which base interventions to be evaluated on both general theory and local practice, include the views of patients and practitioners from the earliest stage, and integrate research with education.

Examples

The potential of an interdisciplinary approach to primary care research can perhaps be best understood in the context of real examples, and two are provided here from the experience of the author over the last ten years, in trials of approaches to care in preventive medicine and chronic disease management.

The British Family Heart Study (BFHS)
This randomised control trial aimed to measure the change in cardiovascular risk factors achievable among a population of men aged 40–59 years and their partners, recruited through, and managed in, general practice.

The research brought together the kind of multidisciplinary team needed to evaluate an appropriate health promotion programme delivered primarily by the practice nurse. The study required strong collaboration with 26 practices which were carefully recruited in pairs from 13 towns spread across Britain, and randomised to intervention or comparison groups. Through this collaboration 12 472 eligible men and their partners were identified by household and took part in the study.

The intervention was based on the epidemiological theory underlying approaches to prevention in general populations and in high risk groups. The tension between these two approaches has been brilliantly articulated by Geoffrey Rose as 'the prevention paradox'.[6] It depends on the observation that variation of personal characteristics within the population tend to form a continuous distribution in which the mean predicts the extreme values. There is good evidence, for example, that the risk of stroke and heart attack rises continuously with the level of blood pressure or weight, with no clear threshold. Individuals at the top end of the distribution are at greatest risk; but since most people have values lying near the middle of the distribution, the stark fact is that the vast majority of heart attacks occur among the many at lower individual risk and not among the few at highest individual risk. Inevitably, the more that preventive programmes are tailored to those at high risk alone, the smaller the impact they can have on the overall burden of death and disability they address, albeit the greater their immediate relevance to the individual patient.

The implication of this for health promotion is that the more everyone takes precautions, the greater is the shift of the distribution of risk towards lower values and the lower will be the overall burden of death and disability in the whole population.

The practice nurses who carried out the intervention received special training, led by a well-known educationalist, and based on adult learning principles. They aimed to achieve a reduction in cardiovascular risk by providing information about the individuals' risk profile, and the changes necessary to improve it, in relation to smoking, diet and exercise. The attempt to shift population risk involved inviting for screening and lifestyle advice all eligible men and their partners in the practice, irrespective of risk. In addition, greatest support was offered to those at highest risk, follow-up varying from annually to monthly over the study year.

After one year, the 'risk status' of those in the intervention practices was compared with that of those in the comparison practices, who were identified on the practice registers at the start of the study, but had not been called in until the end.

The results did suggest that the intervention had been moderately successful in 'unloading the dice'. Overall, there was a 12% reduction in the Dundee Risk Score which, if maintained, might indicate a reduction of about 788 myocardial infarctions and 853 deaths from coronary heart disease in British men age 40–59 years during each year; that is, about 8% of all such events in this group. The greatest reduction in risk was among those at highest risk. The parallel cost-effectiveness study estimated that the costs of running the programme in a four-partner practice were about £58k per annum, requiring almost two nurses full-time to achieve the results of this programme.

During the study, and despite previous research showing no evidence that screening for multiple cardiovascular risks was effective in reducing them in general practice, the government introduced into general practice a health promotion package based on this idea. This package offered a maximum of £8300, plus a contribution to practice nurse salaries, for the whole range of health promotion activities. A workshop on preventing heart disease, the British Family Heart Study (BFHS) and its sister study, Oxcheck, co-ordinated by the National Heart Forum for Coronary Heart Disease Prevention, subsequently contributed to the revision of this 'health promotion package' and to a move towards an approach to disease prevention that would be more clearly based on evidence and more acceptable to the profession.[5] In particular, it led to constructive discussion about the place of general practice within a wider public health strategy for health promotion, and of the GP's particular responsibility for monitoring and intervening with those at highest risk.

This study provides a good example of the power of epidemiologically driven research, through multidisciplinary research teams, to inform important debates about the organisation and resourcing of general practice activity – here the delivery of preventive care. However, it also raises important issues.

In interpreting the implications of the results, a potential 8% decline in coronary events is encouraging in public health terms. However, when the studies were first published, the overall potential public health benefits may have been underestimated because of unrealistic expectations extrapolated from the expected outcome of treating established disease in the few, rather than reducing risk in the many. Clinical academics in general practice have a responsibility to educate medical students and GPs in the interpretation of the epidemiological concepts underlying preventive medicine in which general practice is developing such a leading role.

Another issue lies in the inability of the study to answer questions about the behaviour of patients and practitioners within the study (i.e. about exactly how the programme was delivered and how individuals responded).

The study was a 'black box' experiment in that, although it depended for success on behavioural changes, it did not involve observation or measurement of the process of those changes, only their inferred outcomes. Moreover, although we are perfectly aware, from our own lives, that knowledge does not predict behavioural change in any consistent manner, this intervention was predicated largely on the unsupported assumption that associations between knowledge, behaviours and healthy outcomes are strong and causal.

This was to the regret of the psychologist collaborator, who joined the study after the intervention had been agreed, and whose contribution broadened the characterisation of participants to include their views on personal health and ability to reduce cardiovascular risk. Broadening outcome measures beyond the physiological allowed us to demonstrate that participation in this carefully managed programme was not associated with increased concerns about present or future health but rather with a reduction in perceived ability to reduce personal risks of cardiovascular disease further. The findings were thus of value in considering the implementation of future programmes and raising awareness of the importance of avoiding inappropriate reassurance as well as anxiety. They could not, however, illuminate how the pattern of results related to the way the BFHS programme was implemented.

Experience of this and other similar studies has led to an increasing focus on the design and development of the programmes and interventions to be evaluated in primary care; an increasing emphasis on unpacking the 'black box' study – where impeccable research design is applied to evaluate a poorly conceptualised and described intervention which therefore cannot be repeated or generalised.

Primary care researchers are now spending more time in developing generalisable interventions to support patients' decisions about risk management and self-care, bringing together the understanding of illness and its personal meaning to individual patients with epidemiological information from the study of populations. The approach involves the perspective of both patients and practitioners throughout the research in developing both management strategies and relevant measures of outcome as illustrated in the next example.

The Diabetes Care From Diagnosis Study

This study set out to evaluate the effect of additional training for practitioners in increasing participation in a patient-centred approach to the care of people with newly diagnosed type 2 diabetes.[7] The hypothesis was that an approach that encouraged patients to identify their personal perceptions of diabetes, its care, and their own health, and to discuss these views with the GP or practice nurse, would lead to better communication between patient and practitioner, healthier lifestyle choices and better physiological, social and psychological outcomes over the first year after diagnosis of diabetes, as compared with usual care.

The training programme and measures of process and outcome drew on previous work including reflection on the findings of in-depth interviews to illuminate the range of health beliefs held by people with type 2 diabetes and their responses to advice about lifestyle. These interviews were carried out by Dr Murphy, a social scientist who demonstrated the wide range of ways in which individuals make sense of diabetes and respond to it.[4] This led to a consideration of ways in which practitioners could be helped to become more aware of the similarity and differences between their own health beliefs and priorities and those of their patients, to be sensitised to the wide range of perceptions people hold, and not to make prior assumptions.

The training programme also drew on the increasing body of evidence supporting the association of particular elements of GP behaviour in the consultation with improved patient outcomes. The elements identified included active listening, encouraging questions, enquiring about patients' understandings, concerns and expectations, provision of emotional support along with clear information, and sharing decision-making. These activities were associated with improvement in measures including patient anxiety, symptom resolution, adherence to treatment, satisfaction with treatment, re-attendance and even improved functional and physiological status, such as improved blood glucose levels.

A year was spent developing and piloting the training programme, and measures of its effects on practitioners and patients, in collaboration with local PHCTs and patients.

The approaches finally compared in the randomised control trial comprised agreed follow-up from diagnosis with or without additional training. The additional training focused on ways in which practices could increase patient participation in the consultation. It comprised 2.5 days over two years led by an experienced facilitator. At an introductory half day, GPs and practice nurses both reviewed the evidence for practising patient-centred care, and discussed use of a patient-held booklet to encourage patients to participate actively in consultations. This was followed by a full day for practice nurses to try out the skills of encouraging patient involvement in care, and a further two half days spread over the year for nurses to review progress together, and discuss their practice.

The measures used in the study covered practitioners' perceived style of care and communication, and patients' well-being, satisfaction, quality of life and lifestyle choice. These were selected from the literature or newly developed for the project. A full pilot among local patients established acceptability, comprehensibility and likely sensitivity.

Questionnaire data were collected at one year, at home visits by research nurses, who also measured height, weight and blood pressure. Simple measures were sent on ahead by post, and others were completed at interview.

A total of 250 people with newly diagnosed type 2 diabetes completed the study which focused strongly on measures of process as well as outcomes of the intervention. Results are therefore able to answer questions about the effect of training on the process of care from the patient's perspective, of communication with the practitioner, and on satisfaction with treatment and about the impact on behaviour, as well as on the short-term outcome measures of blood glucose control, cardiovascular risk, and well-being and quality of life.[8]

Patients attending trained practice teams, compared with those receiving routine care, reported better communication with their doctors, higher treatment satisfaction and greater well-being. However, their weight gain was significantly greater, as were their lipids, while knowledge scores were lower.

The findings suggest greater attention to the process of the consultation and less to preventive care among trained practitioners. At formal feedback sessions with patients and practitioners, there was strong endorsement of the general approach and its contribution to well-being. The study has important implications for those committed to achieving the benefits of patient-centred consulting; the focus on disease management should not be lost in the attention paid to the unique experience of illness in each patient.

Towards a relevant research base for general practice

These examples of developing trial methodology for general practice reflect early attempts to use the methods of epidemiology, alongside the methods of the social sciences, to integrate the biomedical and psychosocial aspects of practice, much as we try to do in each consultation. This approach places the importance of the patient's experience of illness alongside the doctor's knowledge of disease, and emphasises the importance of studying the effects of interventions on behaviour (of PHCTs and patients) as well as on risk markers or morbidity and mortality alone.

There is much still to do in developing this methodology, and in any case, not all that is important will ever be measurable. Indeed, randomised controlled trials are but one of the methodologies underpinning the research base of, and education for, whole-person practice.

Other important and sometimes undervalued aspects include simple reflection by the practitioner on individual cases, with consideration of the feelings they engender, and qualitative analyses of in-depth interviews in order to understand better the range of concepts in the world (rather than simply to count the number of people who hold one's own).[9,10] It is as important to consider how young practitioners learn and maintain excellent professional behaviours as it is to understand how to help patients choose healthy lifestyles: there is plenty to do for all practitioners in developing a relevant research base for general medical practice and we should not be afraid to take the time necessary to do it.

Summary

- Research in general practice must respect and help to integrate the long tradition of medical care of individuals in the context of society with newer population-based approaches, and the tradition of the personal physician with the rise of team approaches to care. Research must span both organisation of care and its delivery within the consultation
- The research wing of general practice is growing rapidly but is still weak; the ratio of clinical academics to clinicians is around 0.01 in general practice compared with 0.12 in internal medicine
- The felt relevance of the research wing to the body of GPs might be increased if the questions asked made clear sense in the light of day-to-day practice

- Clinical academics are central to the posing of such questions but cannot answer them alone
- A range of disciplines spanning the social and behavioural sciences, health economics, statistics and epidemiology are needed to inform the cost-effective care of patients
- Multidisciplinary research teams can contribute as powerfully to research as the primary healthcare team can to practice
- Early attempts to integrate the biomedical and psychosocial aspects of practice in research demonstrates the power of this approach and emphasises the importance of studying the effects of interventions on behaviour and perceptions of GPs and patients as well as on risk markers, morbidity or mortality

Acknowledgements

This chapter draws on the author's inaugural lecture in the University of Southampton 1996. Nigel Oswald and John Howie kindly gave me some good ideas, for which I am grateful.

References

1 Fox T (1965) The purposes of medicine. *Lancet,* **ii**, 80–5.
Harveian orations are often splendid. This inspirational piece remains completely relevant today.

2 Heath I (1995) *The mystery of general practice.* John Fry Trust Fellowship. Nuffield Provincial Hospital Trust, London.
A timely review of the place of '*Caritas*' in general practice.

3 McWhinney I R (1996) The importance of being different. *British Journal of General Practice,* **46:**433–6.
The William Pickles Lecture of the Royal College of General Practitioners 1996; from one of the leaders of liberal thought in our profession, the Professor Emeritus, Centre for Studies in Family Medicine, University of Western Ontario, Canada.

4 Murphy E (1993) *Lay health concepts, social context and response to advice about lifestyle* (doctoral dissertation). University of Southampton. Unpublished.
In-depth interviews with patients with diabetes. Excerpts can be found in Murphy E and Kinmonth A-L (1995) No symptoms, no problems: patients' understandings of diabetes and their implications for response to advice about lifestyle. *Family Practice*, **13**:184–92.

5 National Heart Forum (1995) *Preventing coronary heart disease in primary care: the way forward.* NHF, London.
A review of the implications of the British Family Heart and Oxcheck studies for preventing coronary heart disease in primary care.

6 Rose G (1992) *The strategy of preventive medicine.* Oxford University Press.
The classic account of the prevention paradox; that greatest benefits accrue to the population when the many who do not 'feel' at risk take risk precautions, rather than the few at greatest risk.

7 Greenfield S, Kaplan S and Ware J E (1988) Patients' participation in medical care: effects on blood sugar and quality of life in diabetes. *Journal of General Internal Medicine*, **3**:448–57.
The first randomised controlled trial in ambulatory care which found that direct training of patients in management of the consultation could lead directly to improvements in blood glucose.

8 Kinmonth A-L, Spiegal N and Woodcock A (1996) Developing a training programme in a patient-centred consultation for evaluation in a randomised controlled trial; diabetes care from diagnosis in British primary care. *Patient Education and Counselling*, **29**:75–86.
An account of one approach to developing a programme in listening and negotiating for the primary care team.

9 Katz J (1984) *The silent world of doctor and patient.* The Free Press, New York.
A very readable account of the doctor–patient relationship which has not become as fashionable as some texts.

10 Stewart M, Brown J B, Weston W W, McWhinney B, McWilliam C L and Freeman T R (1995) *Patient-centred medicine; transforming the clinical method.* Sage, Thousand Oaks.
An excellent start at integrating the management of illness experience with disease from Ian McWhinney's group, now ably led by Moira Stewart.

9

Medical schools: a poor preparation for general practice

David Metcalfe

Outline

This chapter describes how the traditional model of undergraduate medical education produces young doctors entering vocational training schemes who are at a considerable disadvantage. This means that much of their vocational training is remedial.

The chapter should be of interest to all doctors in reflecting on their undergraduate training but will be of particular relevance to those just graduating, particularly those planning to become GP registrars. It will also have great relevance to all those involved in undergraduate teaching as well as those involved with vocational training, such as course organisers and GP trainers.

Introduction

Nearly every doctor, asked about his or her feelings on starting the first house job, remembers bewilderment and anger that the previous five or six years' education had done so little to equip the new graduate for the job to be done. Most of those entering general practice before the coming of vocational training in the 1970s were even less well equipped for that clinical discipline. When vocational training was instituted, therefore, those providing it found that much of what they had to teach was remedial! Until very recently, and then only in some UK medical schools, little has changed, so that a considerable amount of the educational expertise and energy developed in the vocational training movement still has to be expended on remedial teaching.

The educational shortfall is evident in all three domains, cognition, skills, and attitudes, and the specific problems are all crucial to effective and acceptable consultations. Effective and acceptable consultations in general practice are vital for the proper working of the health service, because such consultation is the fundamental transaction at the interface between the population and its medical care providers. Broadly speaking, these problems are a lack of clinical logic, poor communication skills, and a lack of feeling for patients as people. An analysis of how conventional, conservative medical education comes to fail its graduates in these ways will serve first to illustrate the achievement of those who largely overcame these problems in the development of vocational training (and particularly in teaching consultation skills), and secondly, to indicate what still needs to be done in many medical schools. This chapter will first address some general characteristics which affect the development of all young doctors, and then those characteristics which have specific implications for general practice and its training.

Deficiencies in conventional undergraduate medical education

There has long been widespread concern about the conventional pattern of medical education. The Royal Commission on Medical Education (Todd) and later the General Medical Council (GMC), in its *Advice to medical schools*, drew attention to the problems of exponential growth of biomedical knowledge without any growth in curricular time, student overload, and loss of balance between the learning of knowledge, skills and attitudes. In most schools, there have been internal reports highlighting the same concerns and, like the national bodies, their recommendations have been largely ignored. In an early draft of the GMC's 1993 *Advice*, the Council's Education Committee drew attention to the lack of progress on their 1980 recommendations and attributed it to the departmental structure of the schools.

As reductionism in research and specialisation in clinical practice have burgeoned, senior academics with the responsibility of curricular design have been blinkered by the excitement of their own subject which they want to share with their students, and their ignorance of others' subjects, which they feel cannot deserve equivalent curricular resource. Curriculum committees are battlegrounds as powerful professors fight for curricular time (and, of course, the money that goes with it!).

There have been brave efforts at 'horizontal integration' – the idea that the students might learn about the anatomy of the respiratory tract at the same time as they learned about its physiology and the biochemistry of respiration, and even that the teachers of one subject might make themselves aware of the contribution of the others. Many of these, however, have been subject to 'entropy': it has been just too difficult to have all the meetings that are needed to keep the teaching in step, and new knowledge in each field has been incorporated without reference to what is going on in the others. 'Vertical integration' too has been attempted, usually in the direction of clinicians contributing to the basic science ('pre-clinical') course rather than bioscientists becoming involved with clinical teaching, but again the pressures on busy clinicians have often rendered it impossible to keep up.

Integration, however, whether horizontal or vertical, is not sufficient to correct the loss of balance or the overload. Students the world over question the relevance of much of what they are expected to learn, particularly in the basic sciences (where the tyranny of detailed regional anatomy commonplace until the 1960s has been replaced by the tyranny of theoretical biochemistry, both having to be largely rote learned). How, they ask, will knowing this help me as a doctor? Indeed, do doctors know it? It is widely acknowledged that few consultant physicians could pass second MB biochemistry! They begin to suspect that quite a lot that they are expected to learn is purely so that they can be examined on it! The idea of an explicit core content for the course, defined by being necessary in clinical practice, is almost unheard of in medical schools, yet that alone would allow relevance to be a criterion when deciding what to include and what to exclude in order to restore balance.

That exams control learning is a truism often quoted on medical school faculty boards, and is usually put forward as the basis for a claim from a specialty for sanctions which will demand that the students learn *their* stuff. Unfortunately, few understand that while summative assessment is owed to the public, to protect them from incompetents, formative assessment is owed to the students and should be a learning experience. The two are different in many ways, but are applied as if they are the same. For example, summative assessment, in that it affects students' career development, must be scrupulously fair, and validity will be less important than reliability. Formative assessment, on the other hand, seeks to inform the learner that he or she has mastered a subject and is ready to proceed, and here validity is more important than reliability. These days, few students fail exams, largely because those who have achieved high grades in hard A levels are both intelligent and well motivated. An assessment system which is directed to identifying a small number of 'failing' students regardless of the opportunity and emotional costs it imposes on the generality is itself educationally incompetent, but all too common. The effect of exams on learning leaves tracks which affect subsequent postgraduate education and training. These include the belief that the only worthwhile learning is that directed to passing an exam, and conversely, that a part of the course without 'exam sanctions' is unimportant, but is enshrined in a wider culture which might be called 'pass and forget'!

In the UK, a youngster takes ten subjects at GCSE level and drops all but chemistry, physics, and either biology or maths; takes those at 'A' level and drops all three; takes anatomy, physiology, and biochemistry up to second MB and then 'drops' them to start on the clinical subjects (of which pathology is learned until third MB and then 'dropped'). This persists beyond graduation, each career stage being characterised by feeling free to forget, and not keep up with, what has been learned previously. Indeed, there is at least one medical school which calls second and third MB 'barrier exams', and its staff are uncomfortable with the idea of substituting the terms 'valve' or 'filter' for 'barrier'!

Lastly, there is widespread concern, both within medicine and in the laity, about whether schools are admitting the right sort of people. The pendulum has swung from a selection bias in favour of doctors' children and particularly the children of doctors who were themselves alumnae of the institution concerned, and those with sporting abilities, rightly held to be too 'subjective', to a selection bias focused only on A-level performance, that being held to be 'objective'. The current method, while undoubtedly 'objective', is very narrow, and has three characteristics which may have unwanted effects. It selects for 'convergent thinkers', because they do better at science in school, while good clinicians are more likely to be 'divergent thinkers'; it selects for people with no experience of failure, whereas failure is something clinicians have to be able to cope with; and it selects from young people whose position in their schools, as high achievers, has made them an élite. It does not, on the other hand, assess motivational characteristics such as altruism and unselfishness, or interpersonal attitudes which will influence behaviour with patients. It fails, quite often, to identify the youngster whose application reflects parental wishes rather than his or her own, and who is likely to drop out early in the course.

These are major issues that pervade medical education and are closely connected to the bafflement and rage that the new doctor feels when struggling to be a good house officer (i.e. one who pleases his or her seniors by application, thoroughness, and prudence). What are the quirks in this system which specifically handicap the entrant to general practice by impinging on his or her competence in the consultation?

Implications for general practice

Faced with the criticism that their schools are not equipping students for careers in general practice, senior clinical academics retreat behind the mantra that the undergraduate course is 'education', and certainly not specialty or craft-orientated training. Many of them, however, really consider general practice as medically unimportant and professionally unrewarding (cf. Lord Moran's famous infelicity 'GPs are those who have fallen off the ladder'!). It is not, as they see it, a worthy educational concern or goal. (At least they do not, as they did until the 1960s, consider that a new graduate has been given all the education needed to enter general practice as a principal. An important corollary of this is that the GMC has, after a titanic internal struggle, abandoned its stated aim that medical schools should turn out a 'safe' doctor, so that schools can get away from the 'smattering of everything' approach to curricular design.)

Shortfall in the cognitive domain

While general practice is just as much a clinical discipline as endocrinology, orthopaedic surgery, or paediatrics (which is why, quite properly, the undergraduate education in preparation for it is the same) the context in which it is practised is different, and therefore the ways in which the knowledge, skills, and attitudes are deployed are also different.

In general practice, patients present undifferentiated problems, whereas in specialist care patients have been sorted by the referral system and will nearly always conform to the field of the specialty to which they have been sent. In general practice, patients enter over a low threshold with relatively minor deviations from their perceived normal health, and so are unlikely to have serious disease; in specialist clinics entry has been over the higher threshold of referral, and so patients will be much more likely to have serious disease. In general practice, investigations are not freely accessible as they are in hospital, but in all but a few cases time can be used as an investigative tool in a way that hospital-based specialists cannot. (That means that a GP must have a good understanding of the natural history of any disease being considered as the possible cause of the patient's concerns.) The problem-solving strategy will therefore be different. In most cases presenting in a typical GP population, exclusion of serious illness is the primary aim. It has been said that the task of a specialist is to minimise uncertainty, while that of a GP is to minimise risk, and this difference is proper in their different situations.

The 'cognitive' domain is often simply stated as 'knowledge' and indeed many medical school teachers seem to believe that knowledge *per se* is sufficient for the emergence of competence. Knowledge of enough facts will equip the student to solve the problems to which they are relevant, they seem to think. This ignores the fact that, to be properly deployed, knowledge has to be attached to a logical framework, has to be prioritised, and weighted for relevance as well as reliability. Hypothyroidism is a cause of heart failure, but should take its place in a sensible review of the possibilities: within the heart there are valves, muscles, and a conduction system which are considered first (not least because they are amenable to simple clinical examination), while outside the heart is the arterial pressure against which it works, the oxygen-carrying capacity of the blood being pumped, and a variety of endocrine factors including thyroid function. When students are taken through such a review they often say: 'That makes it simple! Why hasn't anyone else taught us like this?'. The problem is compounded by the mindset of some teachers, still thinking the way they were taught in order to pass the Member of the Royal College of Physicians exam (MRCP), making lists of possibilities. Thus, faced with a patient who is confused, and therefore in brain failure, they tend to demand from the student a list of known causes of confusion like the one they would have had to present to their MRCP examiner, rather than a review of what the brain needs to work properly, from which hypotheses could be generated and tests of them devised and prioritised. The former method is only as good as the list of causes remembered while the latter can theoretically 'diagnose' a condition never before heard of, along the lines of 'Well, something must be interfering with the supply of ...'. Of course, the latter approach falls foul of the 'pass and forget' culture, students objecting 'But that was pre-clinical stuff ...!'.

Students are still instructed that a doctor should 'always take a complete history' and 'do a full physical examination', and are given a formal list of headings under which these tasks should be done. There are four reasons why this is bad advice. First, it is a downright lie: their instructor *never* does so. Secondly, the neurological examination done by a general physician would be quite different from that done by a neurologist (for the good reason that they are doing their examinations with different goals in mind). Thirdly, there is no such thing as a 'complete' history; what the instructor usually means is that questions must be asked under a rigid list of categories (PC, HPC, PMH, FH, SH, etc.), regardless of the fact that in some cases, PMH (previous medical history) is of vital importance while in others it is irrelevant. Lastly, it is unscientific to collect a dataset except to erect, and then test, hypotheses. Indeed, to collect a standard dataset and only then begin to interpret it is *inductive* thinking: the real diagnostic process is not inductive, it is *hypothetico-deductive.*

An uncritically amassed dataset provides not only data overload, in which something important can be missed, but lack of focus such that thinking cannot begin until the prescribed items have been obtained.

The instructor, no doubt an excellent clinician, takes the first few facts offered and then asks very focused questions and does specific items of examination to test the hypotheses that have flashed into mind. The students observe the gap between what they are told to do and what the instructor does, and become cynical, while at the same time deciding that large datasets, however irrelevant, get good marks. In later life they will feel ashamed of 'letting the great white chief' down by not getting complete histories and doing full physicals, and make excuses about 'taking short cuts', when in fact what they are doing is much more scientific.

Clinical teaching is directed almost exclusively at diagnosis, on the somewhat specious grounds that unless you have made a diagnosis you cannot decide how to deal with the problem presented. The reality probably has more to do with diagnosis being the central mystery of the craft, the one thing no other health workers are supposed to do. But when one objects that what matters to the patient is the treatment of the disease or the management of the illness, one is told that junior doctors do not have to make treatment decisions and by the time they do, the treatment will have changed anyway! Apart from the fact that most of what passes for diagnoses are in fact syndrome labels, they rarely take note of the *illness* (that is, the patient's subjective experience of the disease: chronic obstructive airways disease gives some idea of the pathology, but not the problem for the patient which will differ hugely between a building worker and a librarian), but it is the illness that must be managed. Again, there are many situations in which action must be taken (collapse, coma, respiratory distress, acute abdomen) before a definitive diagnosis can be made, and a young doctor often feels guilty at doing so. On one 'grand rounds', registrars were praised for their scientific rigour when they had not administered anti-tuberculous drugs for a patient with cavitating lung disease because all tests for TB had been negative: it was a pity that when she died, untreated, it *was* TB! The failure to spend enough time on teaching treatment and management is closely related to the fact that in the teaching hospital carefully selected patients, dependent in a very controlled environment, non-autonomous and separated from their normal physical and social circumstances, are simply given the 'best buy' treatment for the disease they are found to have: once the diagnosis was known, the choice of treatment was automatic.

The value system attached to diagnosis is highly reflective of the teaching hospital culture: it is unforgivable to 'miss' the diagnosis of a condition, however rare or esoteric, but merely unfortunate to fail to exclude a common condition. Indeed, vastly expensive and sometimes dangerously invasive investigations are undertaken in the hunt for a rarity, on the grounds that 'there was once a case where ...' After two years in the basic sciences course in laboratories where certainty was attainable, often to amazing degrees of precision, the student goes onto the wards of a teaching hospital where high certainty in diagnosis (in highly selected cases) is also the cultural value. To make a 'clever' diagnosis (either an early one of a common illness, or one of a rare disease) gains much kudos. To get negative results from investigations is just disappointing, except of course for the patient. In fact, reliable exclusion of an illness is often intellectually more challenging than its diagnosis, since many diagnoses are made, very rapidly, on pattern recognition alone! But when the doctor is concerned for the patient *as a person*, he or she will be glad to be able to exclude something nasty, however clever a diagnosis it would have been. However, by not addressing the intellectual process of diagnosis explicitly, students exposed in hospital to the first are handicapped when they enter general practice and need to change strategy. Moreover, the hunt for precision, and particularly in today's short in-patient stays, generates an intolerance of uncertainty which in turn justifies intensive investigation. These are not conducive to learning to manage uncertainty, whether in specialist or general practice, yet uncertainty is the common condition of mankind!

In the cognitive domain, therefore, the lack of explicit teaching of clinical logic, the failure to define the aims of problem solving, the imbalance between teaching diagnosis and treatment, the imposition of the 'complete history and physical' shibboleth and the culture of high certainty constrain the intellectual processes of medicine in all qualifying doctors, but pose particular problems for those going on into general practice.

Shortfalls in the skills domain

In all clinical practice the central skill is communication, as study after study and report after report have shown. Essentially, medical care is a partnership between doctor and patient, the currency of that partnership being the exchange of information. Each evaluates the other's communication in terms of reliability (Do you trust it?) and relevance (Does this help?). There are several categories of information, of which perhaps three are crucial. *Factual information* must be accurate and understandable if the doctor is to be able to make (or exclude) a diagnosis and the patient is to believe the doctor. *Feelings* will affect each partner's reaction to the other and the process, and must be honestly transmitted and perceptively received, whether verbally or non-verbally. The *context* of the presentation must be explained and accepted for, on the patient's side, factors such as time, work, home, and life experience will colour what is presented and the way it is presented, while on the doctor's side, response will be affected by the services available. Facts, feelings, and context should be exchanged in all clinical practice, but in specialist practice often are not. In general practice, however, they must be.

Until relatively recently, no attention was paid formally to teaching communication skills, and even now this is usually only done under the auspices of Departments of General Practice or Psychiatry. To many clinical teachers, 'communication' is one way, the acquisition of good data by history-taking, rather than two way, responding to the patient's curiosity and anxiety by giving information too. Little or no attention is paid to feelings or context. Students are rarely watched while taking histories so that their performance is judged on the extent to which they got some data in each of the predetermined categories, and that it corresponded to that available to the instructor from his own interaction with the patient (or someone else's as recorded in the notes). Students often experience presenting a significantly different history from that available to the instructor, and the assumption (often on both sides) is that it is theirs that is wrong. In fact, because they are perceived as 'more human' and less powerful, theirs is often better. Whether they asked open-ended questions or closed, whether they were courteous or brusque, considerate and responsive or thoughtless and controlling, is not known by the instructor if he or she has not watched the process, yet these are important factors both with regard to the reliability of the data collected and the likelihood of the patient accepting the diagnosis and co-operating with the treatment.

Told that they must 'always take a complete history', students find that it takes a long time, and begin to feel pressured. Ask students 'what is most difficult about taking a history?' and four out of five will say 'Keeping the patient to the point'. One student, asked for an example of the difficulties he had encountered in this respect, complained that a patient wanted to talk at length about his hobby. 'Which was?' 'Model engineering' 'And the diagnosis?' 'Rheumatoid arthritis ... oh, I see'! What they seek, of course, is *control.* The agenda must be theirs.

Ostensibly, this is about time, and them not having time for the patient to 'rabbit on', despite the fact that the 'rabbiting' is seldom irrelevant to the patient, as in the model engineer quoted above. But in reality it is about more subtle things. Given the freedom to have some of the agenda, a patient might move the consultation onto unsafe ground or unknown territory. A gynaecological registrar was taking a (very ill-organised) history from a woman whose menses were out of order. Sensing his difficulty in making any sense of it, she tried to help: 'Could it be to do with sex, doctor?' she asked. A look of horror crossed his face. 'Tell me about your bowels' he said! There are other minefields into which a patient could lure an unwary doctor. As well as areas about which the doctor is ignorant, there are others in which he or she is emotionally vulnerable.

In most medical schools no one helps students with their emotional reactions to the suffering they encounter. Relatively young, immature and inexperienced students have to interact with patients who are dying, in pain, frightened or angry, patients whose illness or its treatment makes them repulsive, at least in lay terms. Think of a 20-year-old girl 'clerking' a patient of her mother's age with breast cancer, and having to watch the dressing of a radical mastectomy wound! Depersonalisation is the time-honoured defence: the patient is not 'Mrs Smith who's had her breast cut off (and is frightened of dying, and of whether her husband will stop loving her, and what will happen to the children...)' but 'the mastectomy in bed ten'.

It is even difficult for students to realise that the hospital which has become their familiar working environment is, to the patient, ill understood, threatening, and confusing, however caring it sets out to be. They have to bridge a gap of perception if they are to understand their patients' reactions, and communicate with them.

Most of the time when doctors are working, they are in their usual, well-understood environment doing the job they know well, and so are not in a state of arousal. Patients, on the other hand, are worried about their illness, what is being done to or for them, and how to cope in the alien environment of ward or clinic. They are 'circulating a lot of adrenaline': there is an arousal gap. This is not the only bridge they must build, the only gap they must be sensitive to. Doctors are high social status, expert, healthy, on their own territory, and at least half of them are male, all concomitants of power in our society. Patients are, by definition, usually of lower social status, inexpert, poorly, on alien territory, and more likely to be female, all concomitants of relative weakness. Communication skills are not just about acquiring data: they are about sharing information, ameliorating anxiety, and sharing psychic pain, and doing these things by building bridges across the power gap (and the gender gap, and the ethnic gap, and the age gap...). These skills are seldom explicitly taught, not least because by no means all of the clinical teachers have them themselves. The concept of 'de-powering' oneself is unfamiliar and deeply suspect to hospital-based specialists. The idea that a doctor 'bargains' with the patient about the treatment or even the diagnosis is dismissed as rubbish. Having learned for two years from laboratory apparatus, specimens in 'pots', and cadavers, clinical students move on to learning from horizontal, undressed, non-autonomous in-patients. No wonder entrants to general practice find it difficult to adapt to vertical, dressed, and autonomous patients operating in control of their own environment!

Shortfalls in the attitudinal domain

While those medical teachers who consider themselves educationally sophisticated know that objectives are set in terms of knowledge, skills and *attitudes*, they are less than comfortable with the idea of teaching them! To some it smacks of brainwashing, others feel that students have a right to their own attitudes however bizarre.

Few can think of ways to influence attitudes or methods for teaching appropriate ones, so the mindset and values with which a student emerges into doctorhood are usually acquired 'by osmosis'. There is equal confusion about teaching medical ethics; some teachers confuse ethics with morals and say that staff have no right to dictate morals (unlike the GMC!), while others purvey theoretical philosophical ethics by means of (heartily disliked and widely truanted) lectures, surely the most inappropriate method for such objectives. Yet, ask a class of first clinical year students whether they have seen patients handled in a way that made them uncomfortable or glad they were not the patient, and nearly every hand will go up. Worryingly, the same exercise with final year students gets a much smaller response, and since they have watched the same staff handling patients in the same hospital it must be expected that they have seen the same behaviours but have now become hardened and insensitive (or as some would put it, 'professionalised'!).

Attitudes strongly influence behaviour, and behaviour should be ethically correct. Ethics are the rules which govern all interactions between people where there is a major imbalance of power and the weaker one must not be exploited. This applies in every doctor–patient interaction, not just those in the 'macro-ethical' situations such as abortion, sterilisation, brain death and organ transplantation, and withdrawal of therapy and even feeding. Breaches of ethical behaviour are most likely to come from doctors with inappropriate attitudes to patients, to the job, and to themselves. Crucially, this revolves round how the patient is perceived. If he or she is perceived and responded to as a fellow human being then the relationship that grows will protect his or her interests. Unfortunately, the pattern of conventional medical education militates against such response. All too often, the patient is a subject, a problem or even a specimen, a case in the sense of a container for an interesting bit of pathology, rather than a person in his or her own right. The patient is seen for only a short time, and then in the strange if neutral environment of the hospital bed. Today's short stays mean that the student seldom, having clerked the patient initially, sees him or her again. (When they are encouraged to follow up cases they have clerked in their own homes after discharge, the first thing they all say is how different the patient is in his or her own home!) By thus diminishing the stature of the patient in the interaction, there is a danger that the doctor's becomes exaggerated. Doctor knows best. Doctor's agenda must come first. Doctor's time is more valuable than anyone else's. If they came from school believing they were of an élite or were told in medical school when they arrived (as they often are) that they are the 'cream' of the university intake, such ideas lead to the arrogance which, unfortunately, characterises some segments of the medical profession. The one place in medicine in which arrogance is totally destructive is general practice, because it generates a counter-aggressiveness which in turn makes doctor and patient working together impossible.

Conclusion

The task which faced the pioneers of vocational training for general practice, and which, unfortunately, still faces those providing it today to a large extent, is to counteract the limitations imposed on young doctors by the pattern of their undergraduate education. These include the idea that a diagnosis must be sought in the shortest possible time regardless of cost, inconvenience or danger; that excluding serious illness is unrewarding, that time cannot be used as a diagnostic tool, that treatment decisions are simple and easy in comparison to diagnosis. In the skills domain a lack of willingness to listen rather than ask questions and of ability to explain are compounded by emotional defensiveness and strategies which preclude or severely limit the extent to which they can comfort or empathise with a frightened, angry, or despairing patient. In the domain of attitudes there is a tendency to doctor-centredness which maintains or even widens the power gap between themselves and their patients, and this in turn threatens their ethical standards.

However, addressing these tendencies in young doctors is not merely remedial education. They furnish the designers of vocational training and continuing medical education with a set of goals which constitute a template against which their educational design can be assessed. These things are crucial to good consultations in general practice, and good general practice is the basis of an effective, efficient and equitable health service, and outweighs the other areas of learning, such as epidemiology or health service organisation, important as those are.

The high ratings that GPs get in most studies of patient satisfaction, however, speak not only of the effectiveness of today's vocational training, of which the pioneers can rightly be proud, but of the resilience of the well-motivated, sensitive, and sensible youngsters who set their sights on medicine in general and general practice in particular, enabling them to survive their medical education and, when the time is right (and the conditions safe), grow as doctors and as people.

Summary

Students find that the values placed on different aspects of their clinical role are at variance with those in general practice and they are discouraged from listening, explaining and empathising with patients. This approach is harmful for all doctors but is particularly difficult in the context of general practice.

Further reading

1 McCormick J (1979) *The doctor: father figure or plumber?* Croom Helm, London.

2 McWhinney I R (1989) *A textbook of family medicine.* Oxford University Press.

3 White K L (1988) *The task of medicine: dialogue at Wickenberg.* Kaiser Family Foundation, Menlo Park, CA.

10

Early clinical training

Jacqueline Hayden

Outline

House officer posts will be more enjoyable and more effective if there is:

- an effective induction to the trust and introduction to the clinical unit
- a cohesive healthcare team which supports the house officer in their learning and coaches them through new clinical tasks
- graded clinical experience with close supervision during periods of rapid learning
- one consultant who takes the role of educational supervisor who practises the behaviours that are expected of the house officer and leads by example
- regular protected time in which house officers reflect with their peers on their experiences
- Trust management which welcomes its responsibilities of introducing house officers to the NHS and ensures that they have access to meals when they are working, comfortable accommodation, reasonable working patterns and effective educational and clinical supervision.

Introduction

Most new graduates view the pre-registration year with excitement and anticipation. They are refreshingly eager to begin their new career as a doctor, yet at the same time they are in awe of the enormity of the year ahead. During the 12 months they will be expected to change their job at least twice, some will change four times; they are likely to have to move house at least twice, settling in to new residencies; they will encounter death, maybe at close quarters for the first time and if that were not enough they will be expected to work almost twice as many hours a week as the average worker, with often little opportunity to take a break for meals and they will frequently miss sleep. If this were one of our patients in their mid twenties we would be seriously concerned about their welfare.

Yet, young doctors are expected to struggle with a series of major life events and continue to learn. It is hardly surprising that these doctors rapidly learn how to 'cope'. It is much quicker to take a history and examine a patient in casualty if they stick to closed questions, avoid eye contact with the patient and ignore non-verbal and verbal messages. It is easier to order a battery of investigations, just in case a senior doctor should need it. The house officer will thus avoid being humiliated in front of their peers and their patients. It is easier to adopt an air of indifference to death than be seen to be emotional.

Sometimes, it seems to those involved in general practice training that half of the preciously short year is spent correcting errors that have developed during hospital training. At times, we ask whether it is appropriate for potential general practitioners to spend time in hospital posts.

This chapter considers the contribution of pre-registration posts and senior house officer posts to general practice training. All is not well with these posts, yet there are a number of changes taking place that create opportunities to improve the experience. As GPs we must work with the key players to make early clinical training as effective and enjoyable as we can.

Characteristics of effective doctors

Much has been written about the attributes of effective doctors, yet it seems that insufficient attention has been paid to achieving these qualities.[1–5] With the imminent emergence of the first cohort of graduates from the changed undergraduate curriculum, attention is being focused on the pre-registration year.[6] The year is about gaining confidence in using the knowledge and skills learned and assessed during the undergraduate curriculum. At the end of the year the doctor will normally be registered as a practising doctor and will be ready to begin general professional or basic specialist training.

Clinical competence and confidence

Effective doctors are competent and confident in clinical medicine. Clinical competence embraces the essential knowledge and skills of the individual doctor that are needed in their current environment. A slightly different set of knowledge and skills will be needed depending on the grade of the doctor, the speciality in which they are working and the expectations of the clinical unit. Included in clinical competence is the important attribute of knowing one's own limitations. A competent doctor who lacks confidence can run into difficulties, but one who is confident but lacks competence causes major concerns, particularly for those who have supervisory responsibility. Competence goes beyond knowledge and skills; it encompasses our professional values.

Competence and confidence are gained through graded exposure to clinical situations. Although medical students will have repeatedly taken histories, examined patients and discussed management plans, it is not until they are on their own, having to take critical decisions, that they really learn clinical competence. House officer posts are about learning how to take clinical decisions. During the early part of any post the young doctor will need to ask repeatedly how things should be done and their work will need to be checked, no matter how confident they appear. Yet the experience should not be mundane; if they are stretched while being supported, they will learn faster and more effectively. All too often, once trainees have mastered a skill, they run a dangerous tightrope of asking it to be practised as part of service commitment to the detriment of learning.

Ability to use evidence, set standards and undertake clinical audit

Effective clinical decision-making and clinical management require the ability to collect and use evidence. The recent emphasis on evidence-based medicine might suggest that doctors had ignored the evidence to date. This, of course, cannot be true, yet clinicians can be slow to change their practice when the published evidence clearly indicates an alternative preferred course of action. Some of the developments in computer-assisted diagnosis may mean that we will be able to interrogate the published evidence alongside the patient. However, more effective practice might be achieved by considering the published evidence as a clinical unit and agreeing clinical protocols and guidelines for the unit. Some house officers work with written guidelines for common procedures, but many do not. A few describe the difficulty they have trying to remember which of the four protocols used by the four consultants on the unit they should be using in an acute situation.

Collecting and interpreting evidence is an important aspect of clinical decision-making, but few house officers receive individual feedback on their abilities. Perhaps the most important evidence comes from the patient. Closed questions and interruptions will yield poor information. When we observe junior doctors consulting we often see this style being adopted, perhaps in an attempt to control the interview and hasten an early conclusion. Much of the evidence might even be removed by the time the house officer sees the patient. Neatly scrubbed patients who are dressed in hospital pyjamas, and tucked into bed immediately limit information available. General practitioners have learned to begin to assess the patient as soon as they walk into the consulting room. Observation of gait, dress and appearance all give clues and help us to focus the doctor's questions.

A third source of evidence comes from investigations. Having reached a likely clinical decision, most doctors will want to use laboratory investigations to confirm or refute their suspicions. An investigation result that seems at odds with the history and examination may reflect a laboratory error and therefore all investigations need to be supportive, not diagnostic in themselves. Clinical units in acute trusts are busy, and there is an increasing tendency for investigations to be ordered before the house officer sees the patient.

This may be cost-effective as far as the clinical service is concerned, but may be counter-productive in the education of doctors who need to be encouraged to think through why they are ordering investigations and how the results will influence patient management. It may take a few minutes to order a battery of blood tests, but it can take many hours to sort out a false-positive investigation.

Standard-setting is an important aspect of doctors' work. However, little time seems to be spent teaching young doctors how to set and agree standards across a clinical unit. Few house officers report that they are involved in the process.

A key attribute of an independent practitioner is that they are responsible for their own professional standards. Clinical audit, involving a clinical unit or an individual, is an important aspect of self-regulation. Few house officers report involvement in audit. Those that are involved have been used to take on a project for the team rather than reflect on an area that might help them improve their own practice. Many see audit as the collection of data, rather than a process to improve quality of care.

Professional values and standards

Professional values are important in delivering effective healthcare. The early clinical training can be extremely important in establishing professional values. Using opportunities to discuss the ethical aspects of patient management allows the young doctor time to formulate his or her own professional code within the expectations of the General Medical Council. One of the most important learning methods is the modelling that takes place between a young doctor and a respected senior colleague. Even if formal time is allocated to discussing professional values and ethical issues, if their role model does not uphold those standards the young doctor is unlikely to adopt them.

Skills in teamworking

Effective healthcare is usually delivered by well-motivated teams. These teams are usually multiprofessional, each profession bringing their own perspective and skills in patient care. It is important that young doctors respect and value the contribution made by other members of the healthcare team. Most house officers will have had experience of teamworking during their undergraduate education or in extra-curricular activities. They may need help to relate patient care to their experiences of teamworking and they will need to learn how to behave as a member of the healthcare team and how and when to lead the team.

Management skills

Such skills are important for all doctors, at all levels of training. Sometimes the importance of management skills for junior doctors is not recognised. There is focus on clinical skills rather than encouraging the young doctor to think how their function contributes to the NHS and how they need to manage themselves and others to deliver effective healthcare.

Management is often viewed as an 'add-on' rather than an integral part of training. Like communication skills, some consultants prefer to leave management training to 'experts' rather than including it in their daily teaching. House officers need skills in time management, effective presentation, resolving conflict and negotiation. They need to be able to write reports and communicate orally and in writing. In order to develop these skills they need feedback on their performance, and they will need to be given responsibility for management tasks so that they can practise their skills and learn in a 'safe' environment.

Commitment to continued learning

Perhaps the most important attribute of an effective doctor is his or her desire and ability to continue to learn. This will include the formal aspects of learning, such as attending formal events; focused reading which relates to areas of uncertainty and general reading to keep up to date, as well as the ability to learn from experience.

The commitment to continued learning may be acquired, like many other professional values, from modelling. A respected teacher who makes a habit of looking up areas of uncertainty is likely to encourage others to behave in a similar way. Graduates who have learned through a problem-based approach will, one hopes, have the skills necessary to remain self-directed learners.

Improving early clinical training

The relatively protected environment of the hospital and the concentration of pathology are important in the education of junior doctors. Even if it were possible to prepare for a career in general practice without spending time in the hospital, it might not necessarily be advisable to do so.

The introduction of the specialist registrar grade[7] and the recommendations in relation to pre-registration house officers[6] are beginning to impact on the hospital experience, but problems remain which are not impossible to solve.

The clinical experience

An effective introduction

Most large companies have a structured induction for new employees. The NHS is one of the largest employers and for most doctors the pre-registration year will be the first experience of working in the Service. Some trusts have introduced a four-day induction programme, to orientate new graduates to work as a house officer. This allows more time to ensure that the new doctor is competent to contend with difficulties in an emergency but it is still a very short induction to a lifetime in the NHS.

There is need for every house officer to learn about the hospital; they need to understand about the support services and the organisation of the trust. The induction to the trust is more effective if it is supported by a written handbook. Some trusts have developed a local area computer network, through which all doctors are able to access all the information they might need electronically. The induction programme is also a time in which emergency skills may be taught and assessed. Many trusts include the resuscitation officer in the programme so that all doctors can be assessed and certified as competent in basic life support. House officers also need to be introduced to the clinical unit in which they will be working. They will need to learn where important items are kept and how procedures are undertaken. There is a wealth of information to be gained in a short period of time. Innovative ways of passing on the information so that the house officer understands the trust are important. Didactic lectures may not be the most productive way of learning.

Perhaps the whole year should be considered as an induction to the wider NHS. The house officer, while being part of the clinical team, could be introduced to all aspects of the NHS, including primary care, health services management and public health. Where their clinical experience interfaces with other aspects of the health service they should be allowed to follow the case through, observing how the acute trust is part of a wider health service. The learning would be more effective if the house officers were briefed before and after their experience and if they were able to share their experiences with other house officers.

Graded clinical experience

The current format of two or, worse still, four separate jobs may not be conducive to a progressive approach to learning. The new doctor is just about gaining confidence when they are moved on to their next post. It is striking that the enthusiasm that abounds prior to starting pre-registration posts is dimmed into cynicism by the end of 12 months. Maybe the pre-registration year has parallels to the general practice registrar year. The early weeks need to be spent ensuring safety and competence to cope with common medical emergencies. Learning will be rapid, but relatively superficial in order to cover a broad range of possible situations. Once the house officer is competent to make an initial management plan for emergency situations they should be ready to move to the next stage.

The second stage should establish confidence in the doctor's role as a pre-registration house officer. They should be more confident to work in a less supervised capacity and should be taking decisions in their field of competence without prior checking. With growing confidence they should establish themselves as an important member of the healthcare team, working alongside nurses and other health professions.

The third stage is about the additional skills needed to move to the next phase of training, senior house officer posts. With the thought of impending greater responsibility the house officer will want to know that they have learned as much as possible from their year. Time spent on routine tasks may be seen as time lost from learning new skills. If this third phase is never really reached because the house officer spends all their time undertaking routine tasks, they become bored and resentful.

Moving posts without continuity of educational supervision can be frustrating. If the house officer is treated as a complete novice in the second post, they may find themselves working through the first and second stages again, rather than feeling stretched and supported as they learn new skills. If this process is repeated every three months, they are likely to feel that they have been used entirely for service during the year. Alternatively, the second post may be daunting in the expectations made of the house officer. Without a rapid transit through the safety phase and checks of competence, they may find themselves undertaking tasks for which they have not been prepared. This is obviously stressful for the doctor and detrimental to patient care.

The judicious use of learning logs should avoid inappropriate expectations of house officers as they change posts. The logs need to be completed accurately and fairly so that as much information as possible passes to the second educational supervisor. There may be merit in encouraging all house officers to spend 12 months in one location. This would have the advantages of avoiding repeated house moves and it will create the possibility of face-to-face handover between educational supervisors. It might be possible for one educational supervisor to take responsibility for the full 12 months.

The term 'graded supervision' has been used to describe the process by which doctors are only expected to take responsibility for tasks once they have been assessed as competent. As they become proficient in an area, they should be supported to extend their responsibilities, gradually building confidence and competence. It applies equally to all medical training grades.

Time in general practice

Although pre-registration posts in general practice have existed for many years,[8,9] there has been increased recent interest in expanding this opportunity. General practice offers a range of experience that is not usually available in secondary care. The pace can be slowed and modified to meet the learner's style, allowing opportunity for follow-up and follow-through of patients. General practitioners have gained particular skills in teaching consultation and communication skills and this expertise should be invaluable for the pre-registration year. For many doctors this may be the only opportunity that exists for them to become aware of the nature and extent of disease at first hand. Many house officers will spend the rest of their working lives in acute hospitals with a narrow perspective of disease. Time in general practice should allow them the opportunity to consider the impact of disease on the individual and their families, and the impact of lifestyle and social environment on disease.

General practitioners have specific skills in making a diagnosis and managing care using the physical, social and psychological aspects of the patient. They use their knowledge of disease and background information about the patient and their understanding of social environment to identify a range of possible causes for the presented symptoms. Through skilled questioning, they then reach the most likely diagnosis. General practitioners usually share their management plans with the patients so that, with a greater understanding of their condition, the patient is able to take an active part in their own management. General practitioners also apply the evidence to the specific patient. Although the evidence might suggest one course of action, the general practitioner, knowing the patient and her family well, might conclude that the patient is safer with an alternative management plan. These specific skills of using information from and about the patient are important to all doctors and they are often best taught in primary care. The application of the evidence to the specific patient is not new to general practice but skills in this area will be important as protocols are used more extensively throughout medicine.

Reviewing the potential of general practice as a site for the pre-registration year has encouraged reflection of the way in which we teach about the interface between primary and secondary care. Opportunities to consider the role of community hospitals and elderly people's homes as intermediate care should be encouraged. Also, involvement in the management of chronic disease, especially those in which both primary and secondary care play a part, is important.

Palliative care is not the sole responsibility of the GP, but experience in general practice does lend itself to greater exposure. This should include working with the Macmillan nurses and the hospice if possible. Diaries and learning materials will help encourage the house officer to reflect on their own feelings during the terminal stages of illness and understand some of the responses of relatives and healthcare workers.

There remain some unsolved difficulties about locating house officers in general practice, such as the ability to prescribe. It could be possible to create a limited formulary for each house officer that could be held by the local chemist. As the house officer became competent in each area a number of drugs to cover the spectrum of disease could be added to the list.

Time in other specialities

The pre-registration year has usually been considered in terms of time spent in medicine and surgery rather than in skills gained. As about a third of all consultations involve psychological illness, it may be more appropriate for the house officer to learn and practise skills in relation to mental health. This could be achieved through a short attachment, but it might be better achieved through other learning opportunities. The educational supervisor could ensure that whenever a medical or surgical patient had a psychological problem the house officer was directly involved. Time could be allocated each week for attendance at a psychiatric out-patient clinic. Psychiatrists could be included in teaching sessions for house officers so that the psychological aspects of illness might be considered.

Similar opportunities could be created around other disciplines such as gynaecology or paediatrics. However, there is a danger that incorporating too many other disciplines might encourage the house officer to experience a range of clinical situations without sufficient depth. This could lead to 'compartmentalised thinking' rather than a holistic approach to care.

The public health perspective

Throughout the postgraduate years it is important that all doctors are aware of the public health perspective. Although we all need to focus on the individual patient in front of us, we also need to be aware of the greater population and the limit of our resources. This perspective needs to be introduced early; in the new curriculum it will be introduced to undergraduates. The public health perspective can and should be included in the educational programmes for house officers, both formal and informal. Reports from SCOPME (the Standing Committee on Medical Education) on the teaching of Health of the Nation have been startling in the lack of activity that seems to exist for all grades of doctors in training other than general practice registrars. House officers need to learn how to give effective health advice, which may need specific communication skills training.

The importance of the learning environment

Junior doctors learn through a variety of different ways. Much of their learning is gained through their formal programme. This will include the regular structured weekly session for house officers and it should also include any time spent on formal study leave. They will also learn through informal teaching, such as occurs at the bedside, in out-patients or over coffee with senior colleagues. Finally, they will learn through observing senior colleagues. This might be actual observation, such as might occur when a house officer observes an interaction between a consultant and a senior nurse, or it might occur by following previous action as observed through medical records. In some instances it might be through a third party, where a house officer is informed that their senior colleague undertakes certain actions when faced with a similar situation.

Professional values will be established through the learning environment during these early formative years. Relationships between NHS management and clinicians are often excellent, but if a young doctor is exposed to senior managers who do not respect their medical colleagues, sour relationships and entrenched behaviour may develop.

No matter how good the formal teaching is, house officers learn from watching their senior colleagues and many model themselves on the behaviour they observe. Occasionally, house officers report that they vow never to behave in the way that they have observed.

Great emphasis has been placed on a multiprofessional approach to patient care. Attitudes to other health professionals are established early. It is therefore essential that house officers are placed in units where there is an effective team approach to patient care. Where appropriate, there should be opportunities for learning with other healthcare professionals and some of the formal teaching might be undertaken by other members of the clinical or managerial team.

Attitudes to effective prescribing and management will also be established during these early clinical years. Units that foster a critical approach to new medication are likely to encourage a critical approach in junior doctors who work with them. Those units that value protocols and guidelines, and regularly update them are likely to produce doctors who place similar emphasis on high quality standards of care. When all members of the team review their work critically the unit develops a culture of audit. That ethos will be adopted by house officers as they pass through the unit.

Criticism is often levelled at doctors in training for lack of enthusiasm for learning. When we work in a culture that values feedback and supports protected time for learning, we usually begin to adopt a similar approach to our own learning. House officers who work on units in which there is no culture of continuing learning are likely to adopt a similar stance and place little value on their own professional development.

Developing effective teachers

One of the cornerstones of improving the experience for house officers is effective clinical teaching. *The new doctor* is explicit about the standards expected from consultants who will take responsibility for educational supervision.[6] General practice has already demonstrated that it is possible to set standards for teachers and provide appropriate training and support for the standards to be met. The introduction of the unified higher training grade has brought with it a range of new terminologies that sometimes confuse. The terms 'mentor', 'educational supervisor' and 'programme director' are used almost interchangeably without clarity of the role and functions that the individual should take.

Pre-registration house officers rarely work on the traditional 'firm', therefore there is need to identify one individual who will take lead responsibility for ensuring that the young doctor is able to meet public expectation and individual aspiration through a programme of experience and learning. There will also be need for clinical teachers – consultants, specialist registrars and senior nurses – who will spend time with the house officer coaching on clinical skills. Much of this activity will take place on wards or possibly in out-patients and will follow the recognised steps of instruction, demonstration and observation.

Both groups need help to prepare for their role. The consultant who will take lead responsibility, the educational supervisor, will need to learn the skills of setting educational aims and objectives. They will need skills in assessment and feedback and they will need to develop ways of recording formal and informal education. The clinicians who take a more day-to-day role will need to learn coaching skills. They will need to learn how to instruct the house officers in new procedures and how to help them through difficult situations.

Programmes for hospital teachers are emerging, but whereas in general practice it is clear which of the principals in the practice takes a lead role in education, this is not always the case in hospital medicine. Bringing together GPs and consultants to develop skills in relation to house officers creates opportunities for both groups to learn from each other.

An introduction to medical management

Focus on clinical care rightly takes priority during the pre-registration year. However, all doctors have to take some responsibility for management; this might be as a principal in general practice or as a consultant, perhaps as a clinical director or medical director and preparation will be needed. There will obviously be opportunities later in the training to gain specific skills, but during the preregistration year there should be an opportunity to reflect on basic management issues. This might be in relation to the doctor's organisation of the day, time management and interpersonal skills. If there is an opportunity it might be appropriate to discuss wider management issues during formal or informal discussions. These discussions might be around the managerial aspects of clinical issues, such as organisation of the records, or, if the house officer expresses an interest, more into organisation of the clinical unit or the practice. The house officer should be involved in discussions relating to clinical policy and protocols and there may be learning opportunities around how the meeting was structured and the possible outcomes.

The skills needed to work effectively with patients are similar to those needed for the human resources aspect of management. Throughout our clinical life we spend time trying to persuade patients to stop smoking, lose weight or increase their physical activity. We do this often with little understanding of how to influence behaviour and how to develop innovation. Learning these skills early in our clinical careers might help us to work more effectively with patients and other healthcare professionals.

The importance of committed management

The success or otherwise of the house officer year depends as much on the attitudes of the trust or practice management as on the clinical experience. Supportive managers who spend time thinking through the needs of house officers are rewarded with more willing doctors. The first week of any post is always a time during which new doctors need additional support. It might be cost-effective to recognise this and reduce non-emergency work for consultants so that they are free to introduce the house officer to the unit and explain protocol and procedures. This might avoid mistakes and unnecessary expense later in the post. House officers should be thought of as a privilege, not a right, and postgraduate deans and universities need to review the sites regularly so that the best possible training is offered.

Attention to security is important. The induction programme should include aspects of personal and clinical safety. Trusts and practices that review safety on a regular basis are more likely to value their staff and to be valued by their staff.

Reducing junior doctors' hours is one particular aspect of the importance of management. Some trusts have responded favourably to the task and found innovative ways of reducing the working time or increasing rest periods. Other trusts seem less enthusiastic.

Assessment

As summative assessment has been introduced into general practice it has become evident that some doctors are lacking basic skills that should have been acquired during their pre-registration year. This has raised the question of assessment during or at the end of house officer posts. All house officers should be assessed formatively during the year; these assessments should form the basis of the educational curriculum. All house officers have a certificate signed to state that they have completed the year satisfactorily. Experience with general practice registrars suggests that educational supervisors would welcome more reliable evidence before signing the statement.

Assessment of house officers is being considered. Most of these doctors will have recently completed written assessments of knowledge. It would therefore be appropriate to focus on skills and performance. These might best be assessed by a combination of a robust report that is completed by the educational supervisor supported by assessment of skills through OSCE or observation of practice.

Specific problems relating to general practice

Although this chapter has been largely about the pre-registration year it has touched on many aspects common to all basic trainees. Those doctors who are working and learning in a hospital as part of their preparation to be a GP face particular problems that need to be addressed if the confident and competent doctors needed in primary care are to be produced.

The balance of training

General practice is the only medical speciality that has just 12 months' training in the actual discipline. Although it is possible within the vocational training regulations to present up to 18 months of experience in general practice, it is difficult to secure funding. A few training programmes do offer longer periods in practice; some of these use the additional time to cover skills in minor specialities, such as dermatology or ophthalmology. The Royal College of General Practitioners (RCGP) has held a firm view that training for general practice should be five years, not three. There is some evidence that suggests that the additional two years should be as a general practitioner with responsibility for patients. It seems that the importance of management skills does not manifest itself until a young doctor has to take managerial responsibility.

Integrated training

The current system of training for general practice is more like four or five different jobs rather than three years of preparation. Many three-year vocational schemes include an introductory period in general practice at the beginning; this is not always easy to achieve if a trust is reluctant to accommodate senior house officers starting out of phase. An introductory period encourages orientation to general practice and creates an opportunity to develop greater understanding of the role of the GP, but it is not a panacea for a poor programme.

If it were possible to start with a 'clean sheet', the three years could be considered as a whole. Skills and competencies would need to be defined so that an appropriate programme could be created. The programme would probably include more out-patient and community experience with less exposure to theatre and high care units.

Opportunities to gain skills in public health medicine would need to be created; this might be as a release programme for part of the three years, using study leave or other activities. The programme would need to offer the opportunity of working in some of the conventional specialities, which are accepted as 'short-listed' experience, but might include new opportunities around palliative care and community paediatrics or gynaecology. Regular contact with general practice and primary care would need to be established. Once skills and competencies are defined it might become apparent that more of the training should be based in the community with release back into the acute trust to gain specific skills. The new opportunities for general practice as part of the pilot pre-registration house officer (PRHO) schemes may create additional possibilities for training that will need to be explored.

Repeatedly returning to a junior role

In contrast to higher specialist training that encourages a smooth transition through the five years of training, general practice training seems fragmented and staccato. Senior house officers who are part of the vocational training scheme find that they return back to the first phase of training each time they start a new speciality. They remain always the most junior doctor on the unit, observing their contemporaries moving to more senior positions, with greater responsibility and authority. There will obviously be new skills to learn in the new speciality, but general practice needs to find a way of ensuring that generic skills are recorded. This should encourage teachers to move the learning rapidly through the first phase and into the second where it can be more productive. This will require considerable skills in assessment and curriculum planning in the supervising consultants.

Study leave

Even in the most highly respected units there will always be a need to take time away from the trust to learn. Unfortunately, more attention is sometimes given to study leave than to the rest of the experience on the unit. Doctors preparing for a career in general practice seem to suffer most in relation to study leave. The system of training, with six-month posts, leaves little opportunity to plan how the leave might best be used. Some districts have recognised the problem and arranged study leave for the vocational trainee on a regular basis so that they might attend courses such as family planning training. Other trusts and specialities have recognised the generic and general training necessary for general practice and arranged suitable courses for the vocational trainees and the career trainees.

Retrospective approval of training

One aspect of general practice training that does not apply to higher specialist training is retrospective recognition of experience. It is possible for a GP registrar to submit evidence of experience for two years of hospital posts that have been completed, without recognising that the doctor was training for general practice. If only one year could be submitted for retrospective approval those responsible for the management of general practice training could ensure that the doctor was exposed to a balanced programme for the remaining two years.

Conclusions

Early clinical experience is important in the preparation of the future GP. Hospital posts are improving and consultants are usually eager to develop their skills in educational supervision. There are opportunities to develop the pre-registration year in a way that will make it educationally more productive and more relevant for all medical careers, particularly general practice.

Summary

Formal learning in the pre-registration year will be more effective if:

- a range of healthcare professionals are involved in developing knowledge and skills
- there are opportunities for skills training with feedback
- learning is based around patients or situations that the house officers have experienced
- teachers have been prepared for their role
- the time is protected from interruptions by bleeps and other intrusions
- there is assessment of the learning and teaching.

Informal learning during the pre-registration year will be encouraged by:

- clinical units that support and challenge all members of the healthcare team
- clinical units that routinely reflect on all the evidence available when taking decisions about clinical care
- consultants who provide a role model for the house officer
- graded responsibility for the house officers during the post so that they are working within their competence with confidence but are not routinely involved in educationally unproductive tasks once they have mastered competence in that task.

References

1 Calman K (1994) The profession of medicine. *British Medical Journal*, **309**:1140–3.

2 General Medical Council (1995) *Duties of a doctor*. GMC, London.

3 General Medical Council (1993) *Tomorrow's doctors: recommendations on undergraduate medical education*. GMC, London.

4 Irvine D (1997) The performance of doctors: 1. Professionalism and self-regulation in a changing world. *British Medical Journal*, **314**:1540–2.

5 Irvine D (1997) The performance of doctors: II. Maintaining good practice, protecting patients from poor performance. *British Medical Journal,* **314**: 1613–15.

6 General Medical Council (1997) *The new doctor.* GMC, London.

7 Department of Health (1995) *A guide to specialist registrar training.* HMSO, London.

8 Harris C M, Dudley H A F, Jarman B *et al.* (1985) Preregistration rotation including general practice at St. Mary's Hospital Medical School. *British Medical Journal,* **290**:1811–13.

9 Wilton J (1995) Preregistration house officers in general practice. *British Medical Journal,* **310**:369–72.

Further reading

General Medical Council (1997) *The new doctor.* GMC, London.

Paice E (ed) (1998) *Delivering the new doctor.* ASME, London.

Index